The
SILVER
TSUNAMI
of
SENIORS

Your BLUEPRINT to starting a Residential Assisted Living business that creates residual income and builds a legacy.

GENE GUARINO

Publishing Services provided by Paper Raven Books

Printed in the United States of America

First Printing, 2022

Paperback ISBN: 978-1-7343153-2-5
Hardback ISBN: 978-1-7343153-3-2

DISCLAIMER

All information contained herein is strictly limited to informational and educational purposes only, and should not be construed as legal, tax, or specific investment advice. Each person's situation is unique, and you should consult a knowledgeable advisor before making investment, business, tax or financial decisions.

This book provides no guarantees, promises, representations or warranties of any kind regarding specific general benefits, monetary or otherwise from Gene Guarino, Residential Assisted Living Academy or affiliated partners. These entities are not responsible for and shall not be held liable for any investment and/or business success or failure, acts or commissions, the appropriateness of the reader's decisions, or the use of reliance on this information.

Investing in real estate and/or business does contain risk. Entrepreneurs and investors can both make and lose money on any given transaction. Like the stock market, poor decisions may result in the loss of all or part of an individual's working capital. Caution should always be used.

This information is not to be construed as a security offering of any kind. Prior to making any decisions to contribute capital, investors must review and execute all private offering documents, including the project prospectus and private placement memorandum. Access to information about our investment is limited to investors who qualify as accredited investors within the meaning of the Securities Act of 1933, as amended, and Rule 501 of Regulation D, promulgated there from.

DEDICATION

This book is dedicated to my mother, the late Marie Guarino. She was the inspiration for many things in my life, for which I am eternally grateful. The goal of our first Residential Assisted Living home was to create an environment and a home that I would be proud to have my own mother move into. Even though she passed before she was able to move into our RAL home, our mission continues for the benefit of others.

Mom, we did it!

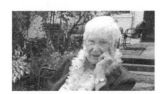

OUR MISSION

Our original mission was to help train, motivate and support others to start, own or operate 1000 RAL homes, providing high quality care, positively impacting a million people.

We Accomplished That

Our new mission is to help others to start, own or operate 10,000 RAL homes, impacting 10 million people.

I invite you to join us by "Doing Good and Doing Well."

TABLE OF CONTENTS

FOREWORD

This book represents the culmination of decades of business and investment advice from a man who thrived on teaching others how to make the most of their lives.

Devoted husband, father, grandfather and founder of the Residential Assisted Living Academy, Gene Guarino was a visionary. He identified a massive demand in the market and set out to create the best opportunity to meet that demand.

In The Silver Tsunami of Seniors, Gene expertly lays out the secret formula for investing in residential assisted living. The senior housing industry is on the verge of unprecedented growth due to the aging baby boomer demographic, and this book shows entrepreneurs how to get involved and build a successful portfolio that will last for decades.

Initially, Gene came to this industry with a desire to provide the highest quality assisted living care for his mother. The senior housing options available simply weren't up to his standards. And so he proceeded to build his own assisted living home in a residential setting where his mother could enjoy her twilight years.

Through this process, Gene developed a business model that not only met an incredibly underserved market but also enabled the investor to build financial stability and freedom while doing good in the community.

His first three residential assisted living homes were such a success that he sought to teach others how to duplicate the process in their own cities.

He spent the next two decades partnering with industry leaders and investment professionals, paving the way for novice and experienced entrepreneurs to follow in his footsteps and invest in the booming senior housing market through residential assisted living.

As Gene used to say, "One way or another we'll all get involved with assisted living. Either we will own the real estate, operate the assisted living home, or occupy the bed."

He lived his life helping others, but he also recognized that in order to have a greater impact, financial stability needed to be part of the formula.

Gene had an incredibly big heart and his passion for people was apparent in everything he did. So it only came naturally that he applied this passion to helping people build the businesses that would care for our nation's seniors with comfort and dignity.

I was incredibly saddened to hear about Gene's passing this past year. It came as a shock to all of us.

I've seen the legacy that he left and I am heartened by the movement he built in raising quality standards for boutique senior living across the country.

Gene wrote the book on investing in residential assisted living. He lived what he preached. A big part of Gene's legacy was helping families build legacies.

The latest edition of this book is the last sentiment that Gene left us with for an industry that he loved so much.

So if you are looking for an investment that is not only financially rewarding but also makes a significant impact in the lives of people, then this book is for you.

Robert Allen
#1 New York Times bestselling author

INTRODUCTION

This book is an introduction to the incredible opportunities in Residential Assisted Living. Whether you are most interested in the real estate investment, the business or both, you will find insight and guidance in this book.

If you want to become a caregiver and you are looking for that type of training, this book is not designed for that purpose.

If you are a caregiver, or a medical professional or someone simply with the heart for the elderly, this book will give you the insight and the BLUEPRINT formula to consider starting your own RAL home.

If you do decide to come to our 3 Day FAST TRACK, Immersion class, you can learn more about that by visiting: www.RAL101.com

THEMES OF THE BOOK

The SILVER TSUNAMI of SENIORS lays out the challenges facing the rapidly growing senior population today. The "super seniors," people that are age 85+, are the fastest growing demographic in the world today.

The BLUEPRINT formula addresses the super senior's housing and care needs. The step-by-step formula utilizes single family homes and converts them into Residential Assisted Living homes. RAL homes are not retirement homes and they're not nursing homes. They are residential homes in residential neighborhoods, and they are being created all across the world today. This book focuses on the US market.

"Do Good and Do Well"
Our motto of "Do Good and Do Well" is the powerful combination of positively impacting others and your community and making significant income for yourself.

Throughout the **SILVER TSUNAMI of SENIORS** I'll refer to the **BLUEPRINT formula**. My goal is to share with you, this step by step formula that shows you how to position yourself to **Do Good and Do Well** by providing seniors with high quality Residential Assisted Living homes and care. Throughout this book I will be expanding on and explaining the details behind the BLUEPRINT formula.

THE RAL BLUEPRINT FORMULA

THERE ARE 2 OPPORTUNITIES IN RESIDENTIAL ASSISTED LIVING (RAL) HOMES. YOU CAN CHOOSE TO DO EITHER OR BOTH.

1. There is a Real Estate Opportunity
2. There is a Business Opportunity

3 REAL ESTATE OPPORTUNITIES WITH RAL HOMES

1. You can own the real estate and lease it to an operator
2. You can own the real estate and be the operator.
3. You can lease the real estate and be the operator.

5 CRITICAL ELEMENTS WHEN SELECTING THE RIGHT REAL ESTATE

1. Location, Location, Location
2. Local Rules and Regulations
3. Demographics of the area
4. Square footage of the home and the property
5. Number of bedrooms and bathrooms

3 METHODS TO STARTING YOUR RAL BUSINESS

1. You can buy an existing RAL home.
2. You can start the business from scratch.
3. You can be an investor in a RAL home.

5 CRITICAL ELEMENTS
WHEN STARTING YOUR RAL BUSINESS

1. The Team – Staffing
2. The Systems – Policies and Procedures
3. The Census – Maximize the Occupancy
4. Filling the Home Fast – Branding and Marketing
5. Scaling – The 3-Pack and the potential to Scale big

COMMON INDUSTRY ACRONYMS

- ADL – Activity of Daily Living
- RAL – Residential Assisted Living
- MC – Memory Care
- IL - Independent Living
- AL – Assisted Living
- SNF – Skilled Nursing Facility (aka "SNIF")
- CCRC – Continuing Care Retirement Community
- ADC – Adult Day Care
- CNA – Certified Nursing Assistant
- LTC – Long Term Care (Insurance)

THE "DO GOOD AND DO WELL" CONCEPT

Some people ask, "is it OK to make a lot of money?"

You may have heard the famously mis-quoted bible verse:
"MONEY is the root of all evil." *Is that true?*

The verse in 1 Timothy chapter 6 verse 10, actually states:

"The LOVE of money is the root of all evil." *That IS true!*

It's fine to make money, especially if your goal is to "Do Good" with it. It is a noble thought to want to give money and resources away and to do something that will have an impact in the world.

After all, you can't give what you don't have.

I love to MAKE money and I love to give it away too. Especially with the motive of encouraging and inspiring other people to do the same thing. If you truly want to give away more and do more you must make more. **I say, Do Good AND Do Well!**

WHO IS GENE GUARINO?

I've been a serial entrepreneur my entire life. I've never had a 9-5 job working for someone else. I got started investing in real estate when I was 18 years old by accident and not on purpose. My reason for getting involved in real estate was simple, we needed a place to operate our business.

It was 1979, I was 18 and Jim was 20, when we bought that 1st property. I was a professional musician and played the drums. My brother Jim, who is an incredible guitar player, and I were operating a music school and recording studio out of a rented single-family home.

I was 16 when we 1st started the business and Jim was 18. The house was in a commercially zoned area of a small community in upstate NY called Clifton Park. We called it, The Clifton Park Music School. Our recording studio and Record Label was called, Saratoga Music Productions.

On the weekends we had a coffee house with entertainment. I was in high school during the week and we were both too young to get a liquor license so coffee is what we served and weekends is when we had it open. That business was called the Gallery Café because we displayed local artists creations in that space. Our older brother George was an artist, as he is to this day. That space gave him the opportunity to share his creations with the world as well. That is also were I met my future wife Mona. She was a waitress at the café. We reconnected years later and we've been married for 36 years.

Over the course of 7 or 8 years, we built the businesses to the point of having over 300 students a week during the day and recording sessions through the night. We even had some of the high school's music teachers working for us giving lessons.

I have to admit, that was pretty fun to walk down the hall in school and tell the teacher, "don't be late for work."

After two years of renting that 1st house we realized, not only were there better properties out there, but we were paying someone else's mortgage instead of our own.

Something had to change, and it did.

After some clear-eyed financial counseling and soul searching we decided to close the business entirely because it didn't fit our "Why" at that time. Back then we *thought* what we really wanted was to be rock and roll stars playing the biggest venues across the country. Instead, we were teaching 10 year old kids how to play the drums and guitar. MTV had just started and playing a musical instrument was something many people wanted to do.

My first investment in commercial real estate was at the age of 25. We bought a dilapidated old church for $27,777.

We did $90,000 in renovations and we later sold it for $305,000. That resulted in about $90,000 in profit for each of us. That was serious money back in the late 80's for a couple of want-a-be rock and roll musicians in their twenties.

If you'd like to learn more about my history, you can read more in the 3rd section of this book.

WHO IS THE RAL BUSINESS FOR?

You're going to get involved in Assisted Living one way or the other. Either by owning the real estate, the business or both. Or you or a family member will be lying in a bed writing a check to someone that does. Right now you have a choice.

So make it a good one.

THE RAL BUSINESS IS FOR MANY TYPES OF PEOPLE INCLUDING:

1. Real Estate Investors and Entrepreneurs
2. Investors looking for a better than average ROI
3. Caregivers and Medical Professionals
4. People looking for purpose and wanting to have Impact
5. Families looking to provide a home & care for a loved one

REAL ESTATE ENTREPRENEURS/INVESTORS

Most real estate investors start with wholesaling or fixing and flipping single family homes. They might be able to make $10,000 to $50,000 or more on a transaction, depending on the area and the details. That entire process and the transaction might take them just a few weeks, on a quick wholesaling deal, or a year of more if there's a major rehab required or if the market changes during the transaction.

The next option typical real estate investors take is "buy and hold" rental properties. This can create $100 per month or more per "door" in profit depending on the details as well.

THESE OPTIONS LEAVE THE
REAL ESTATE ENTREPRENEUR WITH:

1. Limited lump sums of cash per transaction. Once the property is sold you then have to find another property and do it all over again. Finding good properties at below market value is getting harder and more competitive every day. The good news with RAL is, you can pay full retails for the property if you need to and still make your $10,000 per month in profit

2. Small monthly cash flow of $100 or more per month per door. That comes with, potentially, a lot of hands-on involvement in day to day management of the rental. If you want to use a single-family home portfolio to become financially free, it's likely you'll need 50-100 houses to generate enough cash flow to meet your "number."

With BLUEPRINT formula, you can earn $10,000 or more per month with just one RAL home. Instead of investing a decade finding, funding and filling 50-100 single family homes, you can potentially make this amount or more in just 6-12 months with one RAL home. That RAL home can potential earn you more than the average 100-unit apartment building can too.

INVESTORS LOOKING FOR A BETTER THAN AVERAGE ROI

Investors can be active, or passive and they can potentially earn 4%-10% or more, annual rates of return depending on their risk tolerance and their involvement

CAREGIVERS OR MEDICAL PROFESSIONALS

There are many people that have a "heart" for the elderly. There are many people that are "caregivers" at heart just like my own mother was. Professionally there are caregivers that would like to own their own RAL home and put their best ideas for caregiving into practice.

There are nurses, CNAs, Doctors and other medical professionals of all kinds that would love to be a part of the solution for the long-term care needs for the elderly. Many of them are feeling somewhat "trapped" in the medical system and are feeling frustration having to stay within the confines of that system as well. They have a heart, compassion and training and they want to use that in a more complete way.

PEOPLE LOOKING FOR PURPOSE AND IMPACT

I cannot think of a better way to have Purpose and Impact then to help provide housing and care for the elderly. As for the legacy opportunity, my entire family is involved in our RAL business and yours can be too. They have found true meaning and purpose AND I get to work with them on a daily basis.

That is an incredible opportunity for me and for them. The homes you create today will be serving and impacting seniors and their families for generations to come. It truly doesn't get any better than that.

PEOPLE LOOKING TO PROVIDE HOUSING AND CARE FOR A LOVED ONE

Most people are simply not prepared for the cost of taking care of a loved one. They will do whatever it takes but if they are not prepared it can have a devastating impact on them financially as well as emotionally.

The reality is that less then 10% of all adults have a long term care (LTC) insurance policy. The other 90% are "hoping" they will never need it and just burying their heads in the sand.

Using the RAL BLUEPRINT formula, you can own an RAL home and have your loved one move into one of the bedrooms there and they can live for free.

That could take care of many if not all of those family care needs while providing you with significant income too.

Here is a Pro-Tip for you. If your loved one does happen to have a LTC policy, keep it. Start your own RAL home and have them move in. Then bill the insurance company to pay for their care. **It's OK to Double Dip.**

WHERE SHOULD I GET STARTED?

START WITH THE END IN MIND
Imperfect Action is Better Than Perfect Inaction...

JUST GET STARTED

HOW MANY FULL MOONS DO YOU HAVE LEFT?

We will not be on this earth forever. There is a limited number of full moons, sunrises and sunsets that we'll be able to experience. **I want to encourage you to focus on the bigger picture and discover how you can leave a lasting legacy to benefit people for generations to come.**

The Silver Tsunami of Seniors is your opportunity to get started living a purpose-driven life. I want you to experience a life of purpose and fulfillment by "*Doing Good and Doing Well.*"

In RAL there is a Real Estate Opportunity as well as a Business Opportunity. When people first start in real estate, they often wonder where they should begin. "Should I start small?"

My response to that question is simple.

"Start with the end in mind. Decide where you want to end up and find the fastest way to get there" If you want significant, long term, residual income like me, I have good news for you.

Using the RAL BLUEPRINT formula, you can start right now, with little to no experience. And you can avoid many of the mistakes I've made, that you would probably make trying to do this on your own. AND you can get there a lot faster. In short, you can start where I ended up.

When it comes to Residential Assisted Living, if you are thinking "let me just start by dipping my toe in the water with a small house and just a few residents," I understand that.

In this case it's probably better to "Go Big or Go Home."

When it comes to RAL homes, starting with a small home with five beds is just as much work as starting with a larger home with 10 beds or more. The difference is, with the smaller home, you may not be able to generate the income you really want. **I say, if you're going to do a RAL home, go for it.**

THE 3 SMARTEST WAYS TO PARTICIPATE IN THE RAL INDUSTRY:

1. **Own the Home and Lease It to a RAL Operator**
   Get higher than market rent with a long-term low impact tenant providing you with better cash flow. In addition, higher cash flow allows you to buy better properties in nicer areas that'll likely appreciate faster than average rental homes.

2. **Own the Home and Operate the RAL Business**
   In The Silver Tsunami of Seniors, we will walk you through how to earn a net income of $5,000, $10,000, $15,000 or more each month from a single-family home.

3. **Be A Private Lender or Joint Venture Investor**
   - Private lenders typically earn 4-10% annual interest over a 2-5 year commitment.
   - Hard money lenders typically earn 10-14% annual interest with a 6-24 month commitment.
   - Joint venture, profit sharing or equity partners can potentially earn 12-18% annually or more.

I've started over 30 businesses in the last 40-plus years. As a result, I know what works and what doesn't.

Over the past 30 years I've had the opportunity to travel, teach, train, and inspire, hundreds of thousands of people around the world. I've mentored thousands of people just like you. The fact is, the reason I am focused on just 1 thing, RAL and Senior Housing, is the need for high quality senior housing and care is enormous and is growing bigger every single day.

The topic is so important to me and my entire family, I've dedicated my life to sharing my BLUEPRINT formula for residential assisted living with as many people as I can.

My last broadcast radio show "Second Wind Success" was created to help baby boomers discover their "second wind" in business and life. Many people don't find their calling or their purpose in life until well after their 1st career. As we get older most people are looking for true meaning and purpose in work and career.

Ultimately, we all want to make an impact on the world.

When you boil it down, we all want a sense of purpose and control in our lives. We want the freedom to do whatever we want, wherever we want, whenever we want, and we want to have true impact doing it.

Now that you have been introduced to the themes presented in *The SILVER TSUNAMI of SENIORS* and the BLUEPRINT formula. Let's address the most important question of all…

WHY DO YOU WANT TO DO THIS?

IDENTIFY YOUR BIG WHY

I'm not going to tell you that starting a RAL home is easy.

But I will tell you it's worth it. In order to make it through the challenges that you'll face in life, you must have a compelling reason behind your actions. That is your "Big Why"

Your "Big Why" will be unique to you just as mine is unique to me. The goal in this section is to help you to start to discover YOUR "Big Why." It's not about having the right Big Why. It's about having "A Big Why." So, let's get ready to discover yours.

10 QUESTIONS TO HELP YOU IDENTIFY YOUR "BIG WHY"

1. Looking to work less & make more each day or week?
2. Looking to remove limitations or glass ceilings?
3. Seeking the freedom to live wherever you want to?
4. Looking for a way to have impact by helping others?
5. Are you searching for a way to help other people?
6. Looking to generate significant residual income?
7. Looking for meaning in life? Or respect from others?
8. Looking for a career that others look at and say, "I wish I'd thought of that?" or "You were so smart for seeing this massive demand and seizing this opportunity?"

9. Looking for a project that will take you less than one year to attain your financial freedom?
10. Looking for a business that can produce income for the rest of your life, for your kids, and even for your grandkids?

START RIGHT NOW – Write down whatever comes to your mind when you ask yourself "why do I really want to do this?"

MY "BIG WHY"

_____

_____

_____

_____

_____

_____

_____

_____

_____

_____

_____

_____

_____

_____

THAT'S A GOOD START. NOW DIG DEEPER.
Read each "why" you've identified and ask yourself, "Why do I want *THAT*?"

After you've written that thought down, ask yourself *AGAIN*, "why" do I *REALLY* want to do that?

This is the hard part, but it's the most important part too. I want you to be like a 5-year-old asking "why?" right after you've given them an answer. Digging deep is how you will get to your true "*Big Why*." Once you've identified your "*Big Why*," you'll be able to quickly determine exactly what you need to do to reach your goals.

Repeat the process, asking yourself "why do I really want to do this?" at least 5 times for each "why" you identified.

People who truly know why they're doing what they're doing don't usually give up or quit. During difficulties, hard times, and speed bumps, knowing your *Big Why* provides the inspiration to figure it out, go around, or get through it.

If you don't take the time to discover your Big Why, your journey will require a lot more effort, and it will increase your risk of failure.

I can give you many success strategies, but none of them will matter unless you identify the passion behind your *Big Why*.

Your *Big Why* needs to be strong, deep, and personally motivating. We all need a passion that exceeds making money. Money is not **THE** purpose. Money is a tool we use to accomplish THE purpose. What motivates you to your core?

GENE'S BIG WHY

My personal story and passion behind my Big Why started with my mom following a series of events that climaxed with the loss of my mom. When I first heard about assisted living years before, my interest in it was motivated by the huge profit potential. After my own mother got to the point where she needed assistance herself, I realized it was really about helping other people navigating this difficult time. This was much more than money… it's about MOM. When my own mother desperately needed help, my *Big Why* became clear.

WHAT ARE YOU LOOKING TO ACCOMPLISH IN BUSINESS?

Success in any business starts with discovering what you are truly looking to attain or to accomplish. It's essential to be very clear about what you want and why you want it. Knowing your Big Why will become the cornerstone of accomplishing your most significant achievements in life.

WHERE DO YOU REALLY WANT TO BE IN 5 YEARS?

Before you move onto the next chapter, take the time right now to identify your Big Why *as best you can.* **Do** *this right now.* Then, think 5 years into the future, and make a list of everything you want this experience to do for you emotionally, physically, and financially.

HERE ARE SOME MORE QUESTIONS TO HELP YOU TO DIG DEEPER AS YOU DISCOVER AND REFINE YOUR BIG WHY:

1. Is it to help a family member?
2. Is it to help others in your life or your community?
3. Is it to have the freedom to travel?
4. Is it to have a reliable monthly supplemental income?
5. Is it to make your family proud?
6. Is it to be respected as a wise investor?
7. Is it to prove to someone else, you are "good enough"?

Think about the positive impact you'll be able to make.

If you desire to do good and do well – you're reading the right book. That's our business motto and Residential Assisted Living is the perfect opportunity to do both.

"WHAT DO YOU REALLY WANT?"

Most of us agree that we all want to be in the "right place at the right time," and with Residential Assisted Living, you are.

Your timing is perfect. You have the next 20 years to ride this Silver Tsunami of opportunity to shore.

Are you in the right position?

WHAT'S YOUR NUMBER?

You have one life to live, and it's yours to design the way you want. The good news is you get to create your own story.

You cannot change the past, but you can design your future. "Whose dreams are you making a reality... your dream or their dream?"

MOST PEOPLE WERE GIVEN A 5-STAGE ROAD MAP TO FOLLOW:

1. Obey the Rules Society Has laid Out for You To Follow.
2. Get an Education. Highschool, College or Vocational.
3. Choose a Career Path and Commit to a Company
4. Work Hard for the Company Until You're 65 years old
5. Retire. Enjoy the Few Years you have left and then DIE.

3 REVEALING QUESTIONS

1. Is this the roadmap you were taught?
2. Is that what YOU really want?
3. If you chose a different path, what would it look like?

MOMENT OF ZEN – MY 1ST TIME MEETING ROBERT KIYOSAKI

I first met author and investor Robert Kiyosaki when we were both in Jamaica attending The Real Estate Guys, Summit at Sea.

He came up to me and said, "Hey, you're the assisted living guy, I've got some questions for you." I was thinking, whoa, you're the purple book guy, and you have some questions for me? That was my moment of Zen.

The fact is, I had knowledge and insight that he needed and wanted. I had the opportunity to help him and I was honored to share everything I knew about the topic with him.

Robert is a fantastic teacher, but few people know he's an excellent student. He loves to learn and to be challenged.

Robert's book, *Rich Dad Poor Dad*, teaches the importance of financial literacy and financial independence. He teaches on many topics including business ownership and building wealth through real estate investing. His book, *Rich Dad Poor Dad*, has sold over 40 million copies. Over the years I've learned many things from Robert and one is, his "Big Why."

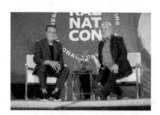

Financial Literacy in Action Leads to Financial Freedom.

Robert is committed to eliminating financial illiteracy and to inspire each and every individual to be financially free. He understands, from his own background and upbringing, that following the typical 5-stage life plan I shared earlier doesn't lead to financial freedom.

To help him accomplish his mission to eliminate financial illiteracy he created a game called the CASH FLOW game.

The first time I played Robert's CASH FLOW game, it was with Robert himself. For me, it was a psychological thriller exposing how I truly thought about business and money. It was incredibly revealing, and it made me ask questions like:

1. How much is "enough?"
2. What am I willing to do to get it?
3. Is money, "life or death" or is money just a game?

The Initial goal of the game is to "Get out of the Rat Race"
So the 1st question we need to answer is, **"what's my number?"**

In the Cash Flow game, you are given a career and the income it provides. That income is "your number." For 1st time players there's a common reaction to the career title and income they've been assigned. Those that are highly paid with "prestigious" careers, feel good. "I'm a Doctor making $100,000 a year!" Those that are not highly paid feel bad. **That is until they grasp the lessons they are being taught.**

To get out of the rat race you need to generate enough "passive" cash flow enabling you to "quit" your "job" or you can choose to continue doing that job because you "want to" and you do not "have to" do it. **The passive income creates the time freedom you truly desire.**

When Robert asked me "what's your number?"

I didn't fully understand what he meant. So, I asked, "what do you mean?" and he said "How much do you need, monthly, to pay all of your bills? The answer to that question is important.

He explained, in order to be financially free you need to generate enough "passive" income to replace your "active" income. Whether you're an employee or a business owning entrepreneur, we all have a number.

There is no right or wrong number.

It's YOUR number just like it's YOUR "Big Why."

What's your number?
How much do you need, monthly, to pay all your bills?

Not pie in the sky like a $1,000,000 a month. The actual number you need to pay all your normal bills and expenses.

1. The House
2. The Cars
3. The Kids
4. The Food
5. The Fun

Now you know exactly WHEN you've reached your goal of financial freedom. The good news is, if your number is $10,000 a month or less, the BLUEPRINT formula will show you how you can accomplish that in 12 months or less with just 1 RAL home.

If you need or want more money each month, you can do that too with either a bigger home or a 2nd or 3rd. There is no limit to how many RAL homes you can have. There are no ceilings, and the sky is the limit. **Take the time right now to calculate what "your number" is.**

Once you know your number you'll have a clear financial goal, and you will know exactly when you've reached it. That feeling is so much better than running straight through the end zone like Forest Gump. STOP just running as fast as you can, grinding it out, with no clear goal and not knowing when you've accomplished your goal.

Unfortunately, many people don't take the time needed to think about their "Why" and they don't know what their "number" is. They just keep running and running and eventually they get pushed out of a job that was leading them nowhere or they retire and then they just lay down and die. **That is very sad but it is very true too.**

After Robert taught me those critical lessons by playing his CASH FLOW game, he explained to me the origins of the game of Monopoly so I could understand the contrast.

Monopoly was originally called "The Landlord Game," created by Elizabeth (Lizzie) Magie and patented in 1903.

Its purpose was to teach the "evil of capitalism."

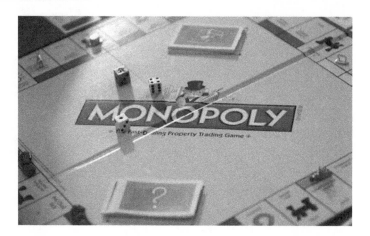

I had no idea that's why Monopoly was created. Did you?

In the game of monopoly, you buy real estate so you can collect rent from anyone that stops on your property. The next step is to buy houses and hotels to put on the property so you can collect even more rent. The goal of the game, and the way you "win," is to ultimately bankrupt everyone else playing the game with you.

Monopoly was created to show the flaws and the "evil" of capitalism. I never thought of it that way before. Did you?

One of the most important lessons in Robert's CASH FLOW game is that you can win by helping other people win. Instead of having just 1 "winner" we can all get out of the rat race and we can do it much faster if we work WITH others playing the game and not AGAINST them.

IF YOU HELP ENOUGH OTHER PEOPLE
GET WHAT THEY WANT YOU'LL GET
WHAT YOU WANT TOO.
Zig Zigler

Here is how you do that in the CASH FLOW game and the game of life. When an opportunity comes your way, if you don't have everything you need to take advantage of that opportunity, partner with others so you both get what you need.

- People with money need opportunities to invest in
- People with opportunities need the money
- People with knowledge need opportunities to use that knowledge

I can go on and on with examples, but you get the point. We all have something that someone else needs. When we "partner" with someone that has what we need and they get what they need in return, we both win.

We can partner in many ways beyond just the financing.

- Learning from other people's life experiences
- Utilizing other people's contacts and connections
- Leveraging other people's time and capacity

Our public education system isn't designed to provide the knowledge or the skills you need to be financially independent.

Instead, it encourages people to fall in line, think alike and work for others. Kiyosaki's game, CASHFLOW, was created to provide the knowledge you need to be financially free. Whether you're a doctor, schoolteacher, or contractor, it doesn't matter. One of the lessons you learn in the CASHFLOW game starts with you answering the question,

"What's your number to get out of the rat race?"

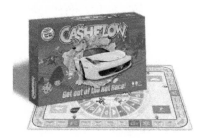

To learn more about the CASH FLOW game, visit : https://www.richdad.com/products/cashflow-classic

One of the many things I appreciate about Robert is that he recognizes the fact that tens of millions of seniors will need assisted living over the next 20+ years. He sees the opportunity and he understands the moral imperative to help seniors too. He is also investing in and creating assisted living communities right now just like we are with our RAL homes. This is reassurance that we are in the right place at the right time when it comes to the opportunities in RAL homes.

THE SILVER TSUNAMI
OF SENIORS

"With the Silver Tsunami, it's like seeing a stock chart 10-years in advance. You know exactly what's coming and how to position yourself today for massive success for years to come"

WHO MOVES INTO ASSISTED LIVING?

The *Silver Tsunami of Seniors* is here, and there's no stopping it. When you offer a solution to a problem that will eventually reach everyone, you have the opportunity to create a better future for us all.

More than 10,000 people are turning age 65 every day, and 4,000 turns 85 every day. As a result, residential assisted living is a rapidly growing industry. This industry is rapidly expanding, and more people are wanting to get into it every single day. I'm looking for people that have the passion, the commitment and the BIG WHY to do something about it.

When my mom needed assisted living, she needed it immediately. This is a pro- tip to highlight, nobody moves into assisted living unless they need assistance.

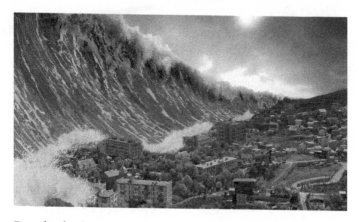

People don't just move in to an RAL homes to have a place to live out their final years. Seniors move into these homes because they need Assistance with their ADLs or Activities of Daily Living.

My mom was living on her own independently for years until the night she fell out of bed. She tried to get off the floor alone and she leaned against the footboard and cracked some ribs. That was the beginning of the downward spiral of her health and her independence.

Her entire life was all about caring for others. Her kids, her husband and then her own mother until she passed away at the age of 104 years old. She was the ultimate caregiver until the end when she was the one that needed the care herself.

This is the DNA for our family business, The Impact Housing Group. This is a living legacy in her honor.

We understand who moves into assisted living homes, and we want to make sure we provide the proper BLUEPRINT for quality Residential Assisted Living homes nationwide.

Let's turn senior's Golden years into Platinum years.

I'D NEVER PUT MY PARENTS IN A HOME!
Many people associate assisted living homes with some horrible place. Perhaps your parents even prepared you for the time when they would need this level of care by threatening to "whack you upside your head" if you even think about moving them into a "home."

Some families say, "In our culture, we would never do that." However, what happens when one of your parents needs professional care, and you are not designed or qualified to be a caregiver? What if you can't just set aside your career or ignore your own children to do it? You may think differently when you are actually faced with this real world situation.

When my wife, Mona, and I decided to get into the RAL business, we went through 104-hours of certified caregiver training in Arizona. Our parents lived thousands of miles away and our intentions were not to work as caregivers. Rather as owners, we wanted to have a deeper understanding of a caregiver's skill and responsibilities. After we passed our caregiver training, it was conclusive; we both knew we were NOT created to be caregivers. **It takes a special kind of person to be an excellent caregiver**.

As an assisted living homeowner, I understand the huge heart the job requires. I also know the personality type and the skill set to look for because we attended the caregivers' training class. Good caregivers are not only great at doing what they do, but they also love seniors and enjoy spending time with them. They invest their hearts into caring for the elderly, and they do it because they want to. They're not working in assisted living homes to earn $10, $12, or $15 an hour. The fact is, great caregivers love caring for elderly during their golden years.

THE LOSS OF INDEPENDENCE

During those golden years, some seniors start needing a lot more help with their *Activities of Daily Living* (ADLs), like housekeeping, medication management, bathing, eating, and so on. But these individuals don't want to give up their independence. The circle of life can be a complicated process.

Perhaps you've been in a position of having to prevent a parent from driving. It's not always easy to confiscate the keys of an adult and offer to drive them instead. Eventually, the plates expire, and another piece of their independence is gone. The Residential Assisted Living business is not merely about making money. There has to be a sense of heartfelt passion for your business.

HOW BIG IS THE SILVER TSUNAMI?

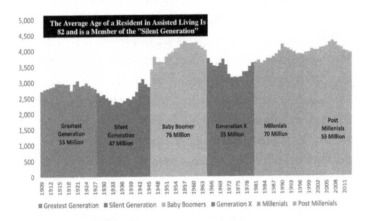

The Average Age of a Resident in Assisted Living Is 82 and is a Member of the "Silent Generation"

■ Greatest Generation ■ Silent Generation ■ Baby Boomers ■ Generation X ■ Millenials ■ Post Millenials

The chart above shows the annual birth rate from 1909 through 2011. The average person in assisted living today is in their mid 80s and they were born around 1936. This was the low point of the annual birthrate on this chart. They are a member of what is called the "silent generation." As you follow the chart along you'll see a massive spike around 1945 and 1946.

WHAT HAPPENED IN 1945 AND 1946?

World War Two ended. Servicemen came home and got busy and had a baby. They said, "that was fun; let's do it again" and they had another baby. You can see the spikes in the chart showing you exactly that.

After the first 2 kids were born, they paused briefly, built their house in the suburbs and went to McDonald's and the drive-in movies. Then they said, "let's get it on and do it again."

I'm paraphrasing here but that is my interpretation of what you are seeing in that chart. 1946 was the start of what we now call the "baby boomer" generation. People born between 1946 and 1964 are members of the Baby Boomer generation.

When you look at the chart you will clearly see that the annual birth rate doubled between the low in 1936 and the peak in 1956. The Baby Boomer generation typically doesn't need assisted living now. It's 10 years before they will be hitting the shore and needing assisted living on masse.

Translation: This business is good now and it's only going to get better and better for the next 20 years.

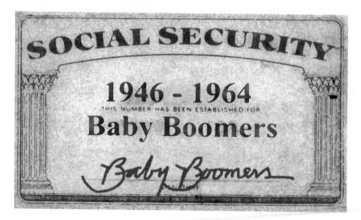

24/7 CARE

RAL homes provide 24/7 care because our residents need to have care available around the clock. Caregivers can either live in the RAL home or live offsite. Both options are limited to working shifts, but 24-hour care is always available.

After operating RAL homes using both scenarios, I've learned the pros and cons of on-site and off-site caregivers. Ultimately, time spent away from the assisted living home allows caregivers the opportunity to recharge, reset, and revive themselves. The role of a caregiver can sometimes get challenging. Essentially, our model consists of a day shift and a night shift. However, a live-in caregiver is an option, too.

If you decide to have live in care givers and they are responsible for providing care 24 hours a day for 5 or 6 days in a row, there are some very important considerations I will share with you in the next section of this book.

These can make you or break you.

THE HISTORY AND THE FUTURE OF DEMENTIA AND MEMORY CARE

Residential assisted living is evolving as a necessary and supportive means of care for senior citizens. Many years ago, terms like dementia and memory care were not common phrases. Today, we all know them all too well.

Years ago, when a person reached a certain age and started to behave differently, they may have been called "crazy." They might even be admitted into an "institution" if they exhibited behaviors associated with dementia-related symptoms.

Now we know that there are over 400 different types of dementia, according to the dementia awareness organization, Understand Together.

Dementia is an umbrella term used to describe a set of symptoms and behaviors that occur when the brain stops working correctly. Dementia results in the progressive loss of independent function for that person.

Unfortunately, lingering rumors left a stigma on senior care. According to the Center for Disease Control and Prevention (CDC), Alzheimer's disease was officially discovered in **1906**.

But the cognitive measurement scales weren't created until **1968**. Today we understand much more about this disease and the care needed to serve those with it.

By **1974**, Congress established the National Institute on Aging that continues to support Alzheimer's research.

In **1983**, November was declared National Alzheimer's Month to raise greater awareness of the disease.

In **2015**, nearly 47 million people worldwide were diagnosed with some form of dementia. Every 3 seconds, another individual is diagnosed, according to The Global Voice on Dementia.

The CDC indicates that these numbers are rapidly increasing. They project an increase of dementia cases to about 75.6 million in 2030 and 135.5 million in 2050.

Think about that for just a moment:
47 million in 2015
75 million in 2030
135 million in 2050

This is a massive crisis coming our way that will impact millions of people. AND it is a huge opportunity for thoughtful action takers like you and me. It all depends on how you respond to it of course.

WHAT'S THE DIFFERENCE BETWEEN INDEPENDENT LIVING, ASSISTED LIVING AND NURSING HOMES?

5 CATEGORIES OF HOUSING AND CARE FOR SENIORS:

1. IL - Independent Living
2. AL – Big Box Assisted Living Communities
3. NC - Nursing Homes and Care
4. CCRC – Continuing Care Retirement Community
5. RAL HOMES – Residential homes <21 residents

BRIEF DESCRIPTION OF EACH CATEGORY

IL - Independent Living is typically an age restricted retirement community. The people who live there typically take care of themselves and do not need 24/7 oversight or care. There is also the "Golden Girls" style of co-housing. A small group of seniors living together and watching out for each other, typically in a single-family home. No caregivers or services are provided.

AL - Assisted Living communities are what I refer to as "Big Box" assisted living. There are typically 100 or more residents in a community. The AL community is usually located in a more commercial setting. 24/7 care is provided and there may be more large group activities available for the residents, as well as on-site medical staff if needed.

AL communities typically charge a "base fee" and then add on additional fees depending on the LOC required for the resident. The additional charges each month can be as much as the base fee or more. That becomes a major concern for the resident and their family because they don't really know how much it will cost them to be there each month. Once they see the real cost when they add it all together, the flat fee that RAL homes typically charge becomes much more attractive.

NC - Nursing Homes and Skilled Nursing Facilities aka, SNIFS, are medical facilities with doctors & nurses on duty and available 24/7. They are typically larger commercial buildings surrounded by parking lots.

CCRCs - Continuing Care Retirement Communities, are larger senior housing communities that include: IL, AL and NC all on one campus. The newest CCRCs being built across the country can be beautiful and have large campuses and extensive amenities as well.

That all comes at a price too. It is common for people to be required to pay a substantial fee just to get into the community. That fee can be $50,000 to $500,000 or more. And on top of that they'll pay additional monthly fees.

The more care they need, the higher the monthly fee they will be required to pay.

For example, IL may be $2,000 a month.

That is to "belong" to the community and have most if not all of the maintenance to their own home be taken care of as well.

When they need more care they can move into the AL portion of the campus. They may pay $4,000 per month plus a menu of additional expenses based on their LOC they require.

If their LOC increases to the point where they need Nursing care, they will move into the NC area to have 24/7 access to medical care. That may cost $8,000 a month plus additional fees as needed.

Large investors, hedge funds and institutions are building these types of CCRC campuses across the country today. The need is growing and the ROI potential is attractive.

If you are seeing those larger campuses being built in your area, you may be thinking, that's a bad thing for RAL homes.

On the contrary.

The good news for RAL homeowners is, the CCRC owners have spent considerable amounts of money to select the best areas based on the demographics and the opportunity that is there.

Your job is to select the right home in the right neighbor within a few miles of that location. You can now move forward faster and with confidence knowing the demographic research and market studies have been confirmed by those institutions and investors, that this is a good area.

Let me pre-answer your question... **Yes** you will have to "compete" with them and that's OK. **You do have a better product to offer**. You're the "fine dining Italian restaurant" and they are the "Olive Garden" They have 200 beds to fill, and you have 10 or 12 beds. You can pick and choose the best residents for your home.

RAL homes are "Assisted Living" in a residential setting. They provide 24/7 assistance with a resident's ADLs but no medical care is provided directly by the caregivers.

THE DIFFERENCES BETWEEN A RAL HOME AND A BIG BOX AL:

1. It's a "home" not an apartment like complex. For most seniors needing Assisted Living, they would rather be in their OWN home or as close to it as possible.

2. The caregiver to resident ratio in a RAL home is typically 1-5 or 1-6. In a typical Big Box community, it is 1-15 or 1-20. At night it can be 1-50 or more.

3. Caregivers in Big Box communities are trained to not get too "personal" with the residents. In an RAL home it is the opposite. We WANT the caregivers to get personal and to really get to know the residents.

ONE, TWO, THREE AND AS SAFE AS CAN BE

The BLUEPRINT formula can be used anywhere in the country. Even in states where residential homes are commonly two or three story homes. Whether it's a small home or big home, a three, two, or one-story home, residential assisted living remains an option.

The ideal residential assisted living home, based on the BLUEPRINT formula, is a one-story home. This allows seniors to navigate freely with less issues. We furnish the homes and make them senior safe. These houses typically don't have to be compliant with the Americans with Disabilities Act (ADA). ADA was created to provide safe work environments for employees with disabilities.

In an assisted living home, you don't typically have people with disabilities taking care of people that need 24-hour care. However, we install grab bars near the toilets and showers, smooth floors, wide doors, smoke detectors, and even fire suppression systems if the state requires them. Even when the state doesn't require them, we encourage all RAL home owners install them. Our goal is to keep people safe, and fire suppression systems help achieve that goal, whether they are required or not. If you have a fire suppression system and your competition doesn't, that puts your RAL home at a higher standard than those without them.

RAL RESIDENTS ARE NOT
YOUR TENANTS

Operators of assisted living homes are not landlords to the residents. The residents in a typical rental house would be considered tenants. They often have children and sometimes even a family pet. Tenants have to sign a lease with the landlord, allowing them to use the home as a living space.

As it relates to residential assisted living, owners are not landlords, and residents are not tenants. There's never an eviction because there's not a tenant—landlord relationship.

In RAL, we have a "resident agreement" that both the resident and the RAL operator sign. It outlines each party's rights and responsibilities. We're providing seniors with a service. Compare it to sitting in a restaurant, making an order, receiving a service and paying the bill. Right about now, you're probably thinking, "What if somebody doesn't pay?" Simply stated, they must leave the restaurant or the RAL home.

In a RAL residency agreement, it outlines exactly how that is done depending on the reason.

WHAT IF THEY CAN'T PAY?
WHAT DO I DO???

Since you are not a landlord to the senior and they are not your tenant, what if I want them to leave or what if they stop paying me for any reason? Take a deep breath and let me share with you the 3 most common reasons a resident may be asked to or required to leave your RAL home:

1. **The level of care (LOC) needed by the resident has increased and the RAL home is no longer able to provide the level of care the resident needs.**

   The resident will likely move to a skilled nursing facility or a nursing home. If this is the case, this should be done as soon as possible for the safety of everyone. This doesn't happen as often as you might think.

   Most residents will live out their lives in the home and eventually they'll pass away. < 5% of the residents will move to a nursing home or a skilled nursing facility because their LOC requires it. 90% will live in the RAL home until the end. **That is one of the attractive things for the families.** They know that their loved one will not be asked to leave as they are nearing the end of their time.

   I know that can all sound a little "scary" to you right now but it is actually one of most impactful ways that we can "Do Good." You are serving the families of the resident as much as you are serving the senior resident themselves.

These seniors are coming to the end of their time on earth just as we all will. Our team can help them through this incredibly important time in a senior's life.

Death isn't like it's portrayed in the movies many times with everyone frantically running around trying to "save" someone's life. Eventually ending up in a hospital bed with tubes and monitors beeping and whirring away.

In reality, it's typically very natural and peaceful. We all have an "expiration date" that we need to be prepared for.

The family will typically be coming to spend more time and to say their last "goodbyes" during this time. They will likely be regretting they didn't come and visit more often when they had the chance. That is sad but true. That "guilty" feeling can be challenging for them to go through, and it is very natural. In the end, they will be appreciative of the love and care that your team provided.

2. **The resident or their family is disruptive to the community within the home, and they can be asked to leave because of that.** It's rare but there are times when personalities clash between seniors in the community and a change must be made. Much more common is there is a clash between the RAL home operator or the staff and a family member of the resident.

Their expectations may be unreasonable, or they may be disruptive even though they may be attempting to be helpful many times. Keep in mind that there is flexibility in the operation of the home, but the RAL home has policies and procedures that must be followed. Asking a resident to leave because they or their family is disruptive happens less then 5% of the time.

3. **Non- payment. It's improbable for a family member to "dine and ditch" on mom or dad.** Adult children move their parents into RAL homes because *THEY* need help.

Not only does the resident need help but the family needs help taking care of their loved one. If they are running out of money to pay for that care, they will let you know that in advance. At that time, you can explain the options they have available to take care of their loved one.

Remember, it's THEIR loved one and not yours. We are not responsible to provide care if they are not willing or able to pay for it. Think about the restaurant example I shared earlier.

THERE ARE 4 OPTIONS FOR THE RESIDENT AND THEIR FAMILY THAT CAN NO LONGER PAY FOR THEIR CARE.

1. They can take their loved one home with them and provide the care they need themselves. As you can imagine, this rarely if ever happens.
2. They can move to a shared room at a lower rate or even another home that has lower rates to accommodate their current finances.

3. They can apply to the state for financial assistance. While state assistance may be available if they truly are in need, it typically helps offset their monthly payments but doesn't cover it all.

4. They can start their own RAL home, and they can moved their loved one into the master bedroom to live for free. Unfortunately for many of these people it is too late. They missed the window of opportunity that you have in front of you with the BLUEPRINT formula

HOW MUCH WILL THE GOVERNMENT PAY?

The BLUEPRINT formula does not encourage owners to focus on government-funded programs because, financially, it makes it very difficult to provide high-quality care and make a reasonable profit too.

Medicare and Medicaid will typically not pay the total cost of a level 3-4 RAL home and definitely not a level 5 home. The amount the government will pay, including the resident's income, resources and social security, is typically in the $2,000 range. The average private bed in assisted living in the US today is $4,300 per month according to Genworth, a LTC insurance company.

If you decide to accept a lower amount because they are not able to pay the full and appropriate amount, that is certainly your option. You may decide to do that from time to time but you should limit that and I'll explain why.

I remember accepting a lower rate for a resident that had been in the home for over 9 years. Her family was gone except for a grandniece that lived on the opposite side of the country. They came to visit twice a year and they were wonderful people. Once their Great Aunt had run out of funds to pay for her own care, we decided to continue to allow her to stay in our RAL home for the rest of her life at a lower rate. She passed away less than a year later.

WHEN THE HEART COMPETES WITH THE BUSINESS

Here was my thought process for that specific resident.

1. This wonderful woman had been in the RAL home for 9 years and wasn't likely to live for many more.
2. With the state's assistance she was only able to pay $1,500 a month less than what we had been receiving.
3. I made a business decision that was supported by my heart, to allow her to stay at the reduced amount.
4. It was the right thing to do and I could afford to do it.
5. She was relieved, her grandniece was grateful and appreciative, and I was able to "Do Good" as well.
   You will never go wrong, doing the right thing.

PLEASE BE CAREFUL IF YOU DECIDE TO DO THIS.

If you do this too often or with too many residents at one time, here are the challenges you will potentially face:

1. You will receive less money making it harder to make a reasonable profit or potentially pay your own bills
2. If you do this, you may attract people that will move in without the ability to pay for more than a few months. They will move in knowing that you will allow them to stay, even at the reduced rate provided by the state.
3. If you do this too often you will eventually develop an unwanted reputation. The reputation of being the home that will "accept" anyone regardless of their ability to pay. Eventually you will receive very few referrals for the higher paying residents, and you will become the "go to" home for those with lower budgets without the ability to pay. That would be a huge problem if you want to "Do Well." The motto is to "Do Good AND Do Well." It's not one or the other, it's both.

WHY MORE WOMEN THAN MEN IN AL?

Statistics show that women outlive men. Often a husband will pass away, and his widow will need assisted living, similar to what happened to my mom. This sequence of events happens a lot.

HOLIDAYS - GOOD OR BAD FOR THE RAL BUSINESS?

Many times, when adult children return home to visit around the holidays, they notice mom or dad looks or acts differently. They may not have seen them for months or even a year by then. They now see for themselves that their loved one has slowed down, is forgetful even simple tasks now seem inherently dangerous. The family is concerned and rightfully so. They gather together and have a conversation about what they are seeing. Many times, this leads to a discussion about mom or dad's future needs.

Who's going to take care of mom if she can't help herself?

If we need help, what will that cost? Who's going to pay for it?

Do we need to sell the family home to pay for that care?

That is an important conversation and it isn't easy to have. Mom needs help and so does the family. That's where we come in. As a result, assisted living homes typically fill a lot of beds during the holiday season.

I'VE HEARD STORIES... HOW COMMON IS ELDER ABUSE?

These incidents, though rare, typically take place in "Big Box" facilities, not in our upper-level model of assisted living. This is because these extensive hotel-sized facilities have hundreds of rooms and limited caregivers. They are typically under staffed and have limited supervision. Many times the residents don't even know the caregiver's name and they typically have no personal relationship with each other.

In a typical residential assisted living home, the resident to caregiver ratio is 5 to 1. A larger "Big Box" assisted living complex is typically 15 to 1 or more.

In addition, statistics show that the fall risk of residents is significantly higher in a "Big Box" due to lower staff to resident ratios. On the other hand, caregivers in smaller residential assisted living homes know the residents by name. They establish personal relationships with their families. The design and dynamics of residential assisted living is unquestionably a more comfortable and safer home-style setting than a "Big Box" institution. The two concepts are very different. Moving into a RAL home allows seniors to receive wonderful care in a high quality, home environment.

THE BABY BOOMERS

Over 77,000,000 people were born between 1946-1964, and they are called baby boomers – I'm a part of this club.

I referenced how about 10,000 people turn age 65 every day and 4,000 turn age 85. Nobody is going to escape this reality.

We're all going to get involved in assisted living in one way or another. Either you're going to own the real estate, operate the business, or you or a family member will be lying in a bed writing a check to someone that does - this is what I mean when I say, "one way or another." In essence, there's no escaping the trend, no matter how famous or wealthy – the silver tsunami of baby boomers is rapidly approaching.

Residential assisted living is the right business for many people in various markets. There are many ways to be involved as well. Whether you are a service provider, a passive investor, or an active operator, there is an opportunity for nearly everyone, including:

- Businesspeople
- Medical Professionals
- Caregivers & People that Have a Heart for the Elderly
- Entrepreneurs
- Real Estate Investors
- Private Money Lenders
- Younger People Looking to Make a Difference
- Retirees Looking for Meaning During Retirement
- People that Can Thinker Bigger and Want to Scale

Remember, *Doing Good and Doing Well* isn't just a catchy phrase. It's a lifestyle that is lived out in real-time.

WORKING FOR YOURSELF

"Many people think that working for someone else is *stable* and *secure and will lead to fulfillment and happiness.* My question is, "who's dreams are you making a reality… yours or theirs?"

So what do you really want to do when you grow up?

DISRUPTING THE REAL ESTATE MARKET

An essential aspect of residential assisted living is real estate. Many real estate entrepreneurs start with flipping houses, single-family rental properties, storage units, apartment buildings, and mobile homes. I know this sounds counter-intuitive, but when it comes to RAL, it almost doesn't matter what you pay for the house you are using. The house's value will go up and down depending on the market cycle in which you live. The key is the cash flow, and residential assisted living homes can generate significant cash flow.

REAL ESTATE INVESTING CAN BE VERY COMPETITIVE

Every new fix and flip TV show brings thousands of buyers into an already over-saturated market. These competitors overbid on similar houses, driving up market prices. It's important to note that there's a cycle to everything, even in the real estate industry – there is a rise and fall in every market-based business. No one knows if we're in the seventh inning or extra innings or game 3 in a 5-game series regarding real estate values.

Regardless, the current real estate cycle certainly didn't just start. It's been going on for a long time. We are in an increasingly competitive real estate market. Residential assisted living bypasses that competition by engaging the real estate market with a business that is driven by an ongoing revenue stream.

CAN YOU BUY A CASH COW?

If you could buy an existing assisted living home that's already generating an impressive cash flow, would you? Current homes are the kind of steady income that we refer to as a cash cow. Buying someone's successfully operating business requires some savvy strategies. First of all, there are very few assisted living homes for sale - this is probably because most existing owners need an irresistible incentive to sell. The few that are for sale typically are not worth buying. Usually, they're in the wrong location, too small, or they charge residents too little. Sometimes they are on the other side of the equation. They are profitable and well-located homes owned and operated by successful individuals – the problem is they may be overpriced.

Our Residential Assisted Living Academy teaches how to build a business from scratch that could be worth hundreds of thousands of dollars in the future. (Register today at: www.RALAcademy.com.)

In addition to the assisted living business itself, real estate also has a market value. However, while real estate has value, the assisted living business can be sold separately.

I once offered $775,000 to buy one assisted living business in Arizona. This offer did not include real estate. I offered to lease the real estate for $9,000 a month with a 10-year lease.

You're probably wondering, "Gene, why didn't you just buy the real estate?" This answer is simple; it was too expensive. The real estate was valued between $2,000,000 & $3,000,000, which would have required a mortgage payment of $15,000 or more per month. You might be wondering why I offered to pay $9,000 per month. My offer was based on the amount needed to pay their mortgage, property taxes, and the owners' insurance. This amount was a lot less than the amount I'd have to pay if I had purchased the real estate. This is the process I used to calculate a fair offer. However, I also reserved the right to buy the home at the appraised value anytime within the next ten years in the agreement.

As it relates to the business component, you must factor in how much money you can make on a $775,000 investment. The financing required an initial out-of-pocket investment of $120,000. The business was earning well over $200,000 in annual profits. That's good but not great.

The seller's income and profit were based on their operating procedures, and it was poorly managed. If that same home were properly managed using my BLUEPRINT formula the annual profits would range from $300,000 - $400,000.

I'm not the only one making these kinds of offers.

With the BLUEPRINT formula, you can increase the cash flow of most RAL homes. The RAL BLUEPRINT formula is the step-by-step process that allows you to do that. One way or the other you have to use the correct formula to operate a RAL home and maximize the income and reduce the costs properly.

IDENTIFYING ECONOMIC TRENDS

We are all potential customers and clients of assisted living. Remember, in one way or another, we're all going to get involved as owners, operators, residents, or by transitioning our loved ones. As a result, it's crucial to have a basic understanding of future trends.

Where is the industry heading? Baby boomers have been driving our economy for 70 years. So, where are they driving us next?

Evidence shows that the answer to this question is senior housing. According to Forbes Magazine, when Jimmy Buffett brilliantly announced his first adult-only community named Margaritaville, it was just 3,000 homes. But over

10,000 people made deposits. Within a year, they had 70,000 people attempting to get in. I wish I were the one who approached Jimmy on that one!

I also read that he is not making an assisted living. He's making an independent living for individuals 55 and older. He's redirecting seniors to nearby neighborhoods for assisted living. Once I read that, I immediately jumped on a new idea. I didn't purchase the nearby real estate. However, I did buy the web domain (margaritavilleassistedliving. com). You see, real estate comes in multiple forms.

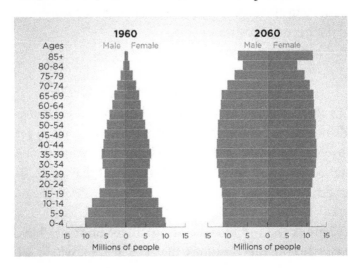

To be a trendsetter or industry leader, you have to think ahead of current trends. Following World War II, between 1946 and 1964, military service members came home and got busy starting families - this created the baby boomer generation. The generation is now a silver tsunami on the rise. With 77 million baby boomers, the fastest-growing demographic is the super seniors, 85-plus-year-old. The worldwide population started quickly spiraling upward since the war. These demographics are more reliable than stock market investments. The worldwide need for assisted living cannot be stopped, altered, or delayed. It's a silver tsunami approaching, and we can see it ten years in advance - this allows us to prepare ourselves. Those of us that see and understand these demographics can position ourselves to profit. While providing excellent service, "Doing Good and Doing Well."

A HOME, NOT A HOTEL

According to AARP, 90 percent of seniors want to stay in their homes for the rest of their lives. Understandably so, why would anyone indicate that they hope to need assisted living as they age? The reality is 70 percent of seniors will need help with their *Activities of Daily Living* (ADL). These activities include everything you do in a day. Getting out of bed, getting dressed, cooking and eating, medication management, and every other aspect of life. Some seniors only need a little help, while others require a lot. Either way, nobody moves into assisted living unless they need help with their Activities of Daily Living or ADLs.

With a Silver Tsunami of Seniors in need of assistance coming our way, residential assisted living is a beautiful opportunity. It's an opportunity for many business-minded individuals to *do good and do well*. Opportunity is defined by how you examine a situation. Is the glass half empty or half full? I choose to see it as half full. I'm a solution seeker – I look for ways to help. Harry S. Dent, Jr is a New York Times bestseller of *The Demographic Cliff*. He says, "the opportunity of our lifetimes in real estate development and investing is likely to be nursing homes and assisted living facilities."

I am not proposing that we pool our resources to build a "Big Box" care facility. Our competition would be Brookdale, Sunrise, and Atria, companies with billions of dollars. These companies are investing in senior housing every day. I don't want to compete with them directly. The hedge funds and publicly traded company's return on investment (ROI) requirements are lower, and they have a lot of money to spend.

Recently, I sat in a meeting with a 38-year-old hedge fund manager. He'd recently raised $485 million with no scheduled investments. So, what happens next? When something comes up for sale, the bidding war begins, and the prices go up. When investment prices go up, the cap rate gets crushed, and the return and growth rate also get crushed. So, big money isn't necessarily smart money, and these companies are big money.

We can do RAL with much better returns with much smaller investments. Our strategy is entirely unlike the "Big Box" concept. I attend "Big Box" industry events 3-4 times a year.

Recently, while sitting with some "Big Box" executives, I had a conversation that typically ends the same way after I explained what we do with residential assisted living homes.

They all said, "That's where I want to put my mom," or "That's what I wish we did."

Instead, they have hundreds of millions of dollars and a responsibility to invest it in the "Big Box" concept. They understand the value in my Blueprint for RAL homes, and they know it's better for their mom and dad. They know how the transition to a smaller care home is better for seniors. Most people want an opportunity to do good and do well, which goes for larger companies.

As a result, they're waiting on us to scale it so that they can buy us out. That is an excellent thing for those of us that have the vision to scale this opportunity.

These hedge fund professionals get paid to raise money and then to spend it. Big corporations like Brookdale, Sunrise, and Atria seek 3-6% returns on their capital. That's a good return, considering that they're deploying billions. If I only made 5% returns, I'd throw up and throw in the towel – thankfully, that's not how the BLUEPRINT formula works.

Part of our training in our RAL 3 Day FAST TRACK immersion class, covers, raising capital. I show students step-by-step how to raise money to start their homes.

However, we do it much differently from "Big Box" facilities. We also do it for different reasons – for us, it's not just about the money. In addition to providing the best quality care, we do so by building happy relationships in home-like settings. So, for those 90 percent of seniors who wrestle against the idea of living in a "Big Box" facility, Residential Assisted Living is truly, home.

LET THE QUESTIONS BEGIN

"Gene, can I do this even if I'm not in the medical field?" The answer is yes; you don't need to be a doctor, a nurse, a physical therapist, or anything else in the medical profession. No medical experience is necessary at all.

"Gene, I own rental properties already; can I use one of them to do this?" The answer to this question is, maybe. Maybe the home you have already will work, maybe not. Residential assisted living is not the field of dreams. The cliché, "If you build it, they will come," in assisted living, this is not the case. Imagine building a beautiful home an hour or two outside of town, on top of a mountain with a breathtaking view. It is likely to remain vacant of seniors in need of assisted living. Adult children will not want to commute that far to visit their parents routinely. Also, absent public transportation, caregivers and placement agencies will not want to travel that far every day for work. **Location is critical in RAL.** Even if you own the property already, that doesn't mean you should necessarily use it for assisted living.

"Gene, how much money can I make in residential assisted living?" The monthly amount varies from as low as $5,000 to $10,000 or even as high as $15,000 or much more.

We understand that you will need proper support to answer your pool of questions when you start a home - this is why the Residential Assisted Living Academy is here to help make your journey faster, more prosperous, and productive. To learn more visit; www.RAL101.com

BE RECESSION PROOF

BE IN THE RIGHT PLACE AT THE RIGHT TIME

"Senior housing is one of the only sectors that had a net increase in the rates they charge year over year, during the "Great Recession."

Generating "passive" income that increases with inflation is one of the keys to being "recession proof."

With RAL there are two ways to accomplish that.

1. Own the property and lease it to the RAL operator.

There are 3 primary benefits when doing this.
- You can charge a higher than fair market rent to an RAL operator because they can afford to pay it.
- The RAL operator is providing care for seniors generating

significant income that's very stable. That increases your safety and lowers you risk even in an economic downturn.

- You can increase the rent you charge the RAL operator each year because they are increasing the rates they charge each year as well.

One of my students owned a single-family rental property that was consistently rented at an average rate for a home in that area.

After learning about the benefits of leasing a home to an RAL operator, he decided to make a change.

Instead of renewing the existing single-family lease, he leased it to an RAL operator instead.

Instead of $1,500 a month with a 12 month lease to a family, he increased the rent to $2,600 with a 5 year lease for the RAL operator.

He also negotiated a 3 percent annual increase and the RAL operator was responsible for all the maintenance. In addition the RAL operator has permission to make property upgrades and improvements with the owner's approval.

1. Higher rent
2. Long term Low impact tenant
3. Little or no maintenance
4. AND, they may even invest money into capital improvements to your property. That is the "Holy Grail" when it comes to buy and hold real estate investing.

To learn more about how you can become a Preferred Real Estate Provider for RAL operators, go to: **www.ral101.com**

"Why would the RAL operator do that?"

Why don't they just buy their own property instead?" To understand their "why" you need to look at it from their perspective.

We all don't have the same motivations and goals.

- Not everyone is going to think like you do.
- Not everyone is interested in the real estate.
- Not everyone knows how to find the property and have the ability to fund it if they do.

What the RAL operator needs and wants is the best location for the RAL home.

They want to own and operate the business of the RAL and they are not as concerned with the real estate opportunity.

If they do not have to buy the property and they can move into an existing one, that saves them time and time is money.

Our *3 Day FAST TRACK* immersion training shows people that want to get into the RAL business how to start, own and operate RAL homes.

It covers all angles of the RAL opportunity as well.
- RAL owners and operators
- Real Estate Investors
- JV and Investment partners

As you can see, you can benefit tremendously from owning the real estate and leasing it to an operator.

"Gene, where do I find an operator?" One of the best ways to find RAL operators seeking to lease a home, networking with current and future RAL operators at the RAL Academy (www.RALAcademy.com) and the RAL National Convention (www.RALNATCON.com). These are both great opportunities for you to network and ultimately make the perfect match. Aspiring real estate investors seek operators and aspiring operators seek investors.

Attending the RAL Academy *3 Day FAST TRACK* immersion training is important for real estate entrepreneurs and for investors as well for a number of reasons.

1. You will learn what to look for in a "good" RAL operator
2. You will learn the best location and what to look for in the property itself.
3. You may meet RAL operators that you'll lease to

Pro-Tip
Find the operator/tenant before you buy the property to rent to them. This will make your life much smoother.

IF YOU DON'T ASK YOU DON'T GET

My mother taught me that as a little boy and it holds true to this day. **Many people ask me, "Gene, how much can I charge for rent?"** The answer is, it starts with whatever you ask for and whatever the tenant is willing to pay. You each have a number in mind and a purpose to accomplish. If it's a win-win arrangement, then it works for everyone.

The short answer is: It's negotiable.

People may decide not to buy a house for many reasons.

1. They may lack the resources or credit to do it.
2. They may not have the knowledge or the confidence to come up with the capital.
3. They goal is to own and operate the business and they simply do not want to own the real estate.

The bottom line is, many business owners are willing to pay more than it would cost to own real estate.

When you rent your single-family property to a family, it is different from renting to a RAL operator. For RAL homes, you can raise the rent. Whatever they're willing to pay is what you can charge. Even when other real estate owners are charging $1,500 for a house, you still have the option to name your price independently. Consider the cost of a steak dinner at the Golden Corral, which is less than $15. The same meal may cost $100 at Ruth's Chris Steak House.

Ultimately, the price you charge for rent or the amount you are willing to accept is completely up to you.

Another benefit of renting to residential assisted living tenants is that the residents are low impact and long term.

Typically, you don't want to lease a property for a short time unless you are in the short term rental business. Even annual leases can be a problem because the home may need some repairs or refreshing and that means you may miss a month or two in rental income.

Given the option, you'd rather have a long-term tenant. The operator of a RAL would rather have the security of a long-term lease as well. So, if you had a small business willing to pay twice the rent while requesting a five-year lease, would that work in your favor? Of course, it would; that's a silly no-brainer question. With RAL you can own the real estate and create a significant amount of residual cash flow.

INCREASING YOUR CASH FLOW

If I owned a single-family home and I rented it out, earning a $100, or even $200 a month, that wouldn't work in my world. I need a lot more income than that. When my RAL journey started, I knew that I could generate $10,000 a month from a single-family home. So, originally our goal was to own four RAL homes. We also wanted varying levels and pricing so that we could satisfy any budget. Everyone has to have their own goals and reasons. Perhaps one RAL home is enough for you, and ten the right number for someone else. We have students who dream of owning 100 or more luxury RAL homes and selling them off to the hedge funds within the next few years.

NICER PROPERTIES = MORE PROFIT POTENTIAL

As my business progressed, I recognized the need for various levels of assisted living homes. These levels are created to accommodate different price points that people can afford based on their budgets. Our first home was a level 3, and our next homes were a level 4 and level 5.

The 5 Levels

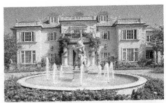

- Level #5 – High End
- Level #4 – Sweet Spot
- Level #3 – Sweet Spot
- Level #2 – OK
- Level #1 – Low End

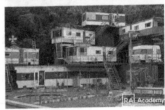

WHAT'S YOUR GOAL?
WHAT'S YOUR MISSION?

The mission of the RAL Academy is to assist, train and support 25-percent of assisted living homeowners and operators across the country. We are well on our way. We are the premier resource for all things Residential Assisted Living.

Visit www.RAL101.com to learn more.

How did we set our goal of helping 25 percent of all assisted living homes nationwide?

That started with a conversation with my wife during the open house for our second home. Mona and I realized that we could move in if we ever needed to. Based on the nightmare we experienced when trying to find help for my mom, we knew we didn't want our kids to face those same challenges. This is why we're aiming to increase senior living quality while helping owners earn meaningful cash flow. By helping 10,000 homes, or about 25 percent of the RAL homes in the United States, we will be doing our part to do good and do well.

LONG-TERM CARE INSURANCE

Most people do not have a long-term care insurance plan that will pay for their future assisted living needs. Most people ignore the potential future reality of needing care and they assume their adult children will that care of them. The thought is, the oldest, wisest, and bravest will manage their affairs if necessary.

Typically, in a family, you have some responsible people, and some that are irresponsible. One adult child may have a lot of money, and another has little or no money.

There are 3 main parts to a LTC policy:

1. The waiting period before you start collecting
2. The maximum Amount per day you can collect
3. The total lifetime benefit in time and money

The waiting period in a policy written 30 or 40 years ago may be as little as "0" days. You apply for the benefit and once approved, the payment is retroactive to day 1. Sweet deal.

Today's policy will typically have a 90-180 day waiting period.

That means 1st 60-180 days of care are paid "out of pocket" and then you start to collect.

The maximum amount you receive is typically $100 per day or more. There may be an option for a cost of living rider as well. That would increase the $100 a day by the rate of inflation or a flat amount or 3% or so.

That means if a policy that was written 30 or 40 years ago with a $100 per day benefit with a 3% annual cost of living rider, could pay out $300 a day today.

That is $9,000 for a 30 day month.

$300 a day may be much higher than you are charging now.

PRO-TIP
You can charge the residents in your home different rates depending on several factors.

1. Their level of care
2. Private room vs. shared
3. Private bathroom vs shared

If your resident has a LTC policy, they probably don't know themselves what the maximum allowable amount is. If you know that amount you can charge that amount and you should. That is unless they also have a maximum benefit payout written into their policy.

Even if they do, you can charge a higher rate for the 1st couple of years and then a lower rate after that to make the money last longer.

If you personally have an LTC policy and you also own the RAL home, you have even more options.

If you do have long-term care insurance, keep it. You can still move into your own home and bill the insurance company for the expense. You can and should "Double Dip."

If you don't have long-term care insurance, that's OK too. I've got a better plan for you. Why spend thousands annually on a policy when you can earn $10,000 monthly and move into your own house if needed? Long-term care insurance is the ultimate asset protection strategy. And that is important whether you have a LTC insurance policy or you own your own RAL home or both.

A NEW PERSPECTIVE ON RAISING CAPITAL

You may be able to write a check, and you may have all the capital you'll ever need. However, many people don't want to own and operate; they want to invest in real estate or business. Raising money for assisted living is the most straightforward business I've ever raised capital for in any industry. Keep in mind that I've been an entrepreneur for more than 40 years and I've done lots of deals and had many businesses.

Many people want to get into RAL because of the high ROI and they see it producing positive outcomes across the country. Many of these people want to invest and they want to get involved in the industry, but they don't want to be hands on.

Perhaps you're thinking, I want to do RAL but I don't have the money to do it. I wish I had the money to do this. Wishing for something isn't going to make it happen. If you want to learn how to do it, with or without your own money, the RAL Academy can show you how. You can do it with or without using your own funds. You can learn more about raising capital at the RAL Academy's 3-Day *FAST TRACK* immersion training at www.RAL101.com

At this very moment, people are searching the internet, reading newspapers, and balancing their bank accounts, hoping to find somewhere to invest their money. The stock market is too risky for some people so they are looking for a lower-risk investment opportunity. As their money sits in the bank, the rate of return is little to nothing. According to USA Today, the average rate of return on a CD is currently only paying about 1 percent. Given an alternative, many people with money to invest are excited to invest to get a solid ROI of 4-8% for a 2–5-year time frame knowing they are making an impact with their investment. You may be the perfect piece to their puzzle, but they don't know you exist yet. This is why you need to be ready to present a professional business plan and have an appealing presentation ready to go. You will also need to be prepared to answer an avalanche of likely questions. This is how capital is raised every day. If you want to learn more about how to raise capital for your RAL home or any project, visit www.PitchMastersAcademy.com.

LENDERS AND BORROWERS

When a bank or an individual lends money to someone, they typically create and hold a promissory note. A promissory note is a properly documented "I owe you."

It's the legally binding paperwork that details the terms of the loan and it documents the borrowers promise to pay the money back. The lender is the note holder and as the note holder they are entitled to receive the payments, according to the terms of the note.

When it comes to a bank making the loan to you, the bank is the one "holding" the note.

- You sign the loan papers which details the terms of the loan and includes the promissory note, and in most cases, a lien on any assets.

In addition, many times the bank will require the borrower to "personally guarantee" the note to ensure they get paid back.

They lend you the money based on the terms you've agreed to in the promissory note

- The bank then receives the payments per the terms agreed to in the promissory note they hold.

In many cases, the bank sells their notes to larger financial institutions, and they get their money back and repeat the process.

The bank's job is to deploy the funds and they get paid loan servicing fees. Whoever "holds" the note receives the payments.

In some cases, the investors may want more than just a return on the loan in the form of interest payments. They may require a percentage of ownership commonly referred to as "equity" or a share of the profits. Profit-sharing means you do not own a piece of the company or property, but you receive a share of the profits.

Borrowing money is usually the best option for someone that just needs capital but doesn't want a partner or to give up any ownership. When you borrow money and then pay it back, the lender is "satisfied" and they are then out of the picture.

On the other hand, if you're lending the money, you may want to negotiate a deal that provides you with some ownership or an equity position. If you do that you retain an equity position, as well as the payments from the promissory note.

For providing the capital and investing your money, you may get smaller return of 4-6% plus a percentage of ownership in the property or the business. This is a good position to be in because, even if the loan you made is refinanced and you receive all of your money back, you are still in an ownership position. In the longer term, you should end up with receiving a much higher rate of return.

The terms of the loan that you will want will depend on whether you are the lender or the borrower. How you approach the contract depends on which side of the table you're sitting on during the deal-making process.

THE RAL BLUEPRINT
FORMULA – THE BUSINESS

AN AVERAGE RAL HOME

$ 4,000	Per Person Per Month
x 10	Residents
$40,000	Potential Gross Income
-$25,000	Typical Expenses
-$ 5,000	Rent or Debt Service
$10,000	Potential Monthly Profit

A "BIGGER AND NICER" RAL HOME

$ 5,000	Per Person Per Month
x 16	Residents
$80,000	Potential Gross Income
-$40,000	Typical Expenses
-$10,000	Rent or Debt Service
$30,000	Potential Monthly Profit

Have I caught your attention?

THE BUSINESS BEHIND ASSISTED LIVING

"There are many need-to-know details about owning and operating a residential assisted living business that you should learn before starting."

LICENSING REQUIREMENTS

I'm often asked, "Is there a license required?" The answer is, "Yes and no." There are thousands of RAL homes across the country operating without a license. You can do it that way, but I discourage it. Launch your assisted living home without taking shortcuts. A license documents that you are operating under state rules and regulations. A license is typically required to obtain professional liability insurance and receive payments from long-term care (LTC) insurance companies. At the RAL Academy we know the rules and regulations required to get properly licensed across the country. The RAL National Association awards you the RALS or Residential Assisted Living Specialist designation. To learn more visit www.RALNA.org

There are a few states that have little if any rules for residential assisted living homes. That is a good and a bad thing. It's easier to get started BUT without set guidelines there is more exposure and potential liability for an unlicensed RAL operator.

As a result, these states have people opening businesses with little oversight. Rules help us to maintain a standard. It's essential to know the rules, so you'll know how to accomplish your goals appropriately. When we talk about senior living, rules are there to keep seniors safe.

On the flip side, they also keep your business safe from accidents, lawsuits, and potential problems. So, if you follow the rules and do it right, you'll help keep your business safe and avoid potential liabilities. Your assisted living home needs to be senior-safe, complete with the proper construction. Your home will need to be physically safe, which may include grab bars, smoke detectors, and fire suppression systems. Even if you go the route of bypassing a license, specific safety components are still required by certain cities, states, and county regulations.

The state will require that you have policies and procedures. For example, you'll need written guidelines of what happens during a crisis. If a severe storm causes a flood and renders your home uninhabitable, you'll need a contingency plan. A power outage can spoil food and affect certain medications, and that's one of the many reasons why policies and procedures must be in place.

Your policies and procedures must include an emergency plan. These plans are called Standard Operating Procedures

(SOP) in most other types of businesses. In the RAL industry, the SOPs are called policies and procedures. These include everything from checking a resident in to the home, menus, medication management, and every detail in between.

YOU'LL NEED A QUALIFIED MANAGER & CAREGIVERS

In addition to safety compliance and policies and procedures, every owner and operator needs a qualified manager and caregivers on record. Each state has their own requirements regarding the manager and the caregivers.

A manager in the state's view, is responsible for the administrative activities within the home. Some states refer to this position as the manager, and others call it the administrator. Either way, you'll need someone qualified according to the requirements of the state and on record.

Some states have meager requirements for managers and other states have much more in-depth requirements. For example, minimum requirements for managers often include:

- Showing proof of being 18 years old or older
- Earned a high school diploma or GED equivalent
- Completing a 24-hour training approved by the state.
- Caregivers may need to be 18+ and "fog a mirror"

I'm being a little humorous there but the requirements for being a caregiver in some states is very minimal.

That's a shallow bar for being a manager or a caregiver.
On the high end, states like Arizona require all of that and in addition they require:

1. Caregivers must complete a 60+ hour caregiver training.
2. Get a criminal background check with a fingerprint card
3. Must have a current TB test and update that annually.
4. And they must receive continuing education annually.

Then to become a manager,
1. They must complete an additional 40-hour state-approved manager training.
2. And they will need two years of experience as a caregiver before getting their manager's license.
3. Arizona has a higher standard than many others. Most states are somewhere between these two examples.

Our BLUEPRINT formula discourages owners from operating as managers themselves on a day-to-day basis.

However, you must understand every business component to be most successful - this is why my wife, Mona, and I went through the caregiver training course in Arizona. Yet, we have no intention of ever working as caregivers.

I'm not suggesting that every owner undergo such intense training like we did. We had no choice because we had no one to teach us the details about the business. We had no option but to figure it out on our own. The process of trying to figure it all out on our own was time-consuming, painful, expensive, and a lot of work.

The good news is, now, there is training that exists to help you avoid struggling for years trying to figure out the business on your own. Residential Assisted Living Academy allows ambitious entrepreneurs to gain years of information in a matter of 3 days. It will enable you to learn the proper way of providing quality care to seniors. It eliminates stress, strengthening your chances of passing inspections. The training will educate you on how to fulfill licensing requirements.

AVOIDING OBSTACLES

Some states have no limits on how many seniors can occupy one home. However, some states impose specific limitations. For example, a state regulation could stipulate occupancy guidelines, limiting one single-family home to four unrelated adults. That can be a problem if you want to make money as a RAL home owner or operator.

The good news is, according to the Federal Fair Housing Act, this regulation is discriminatory.

States cannot legally prevent un-related seniors from living together. This is why the Residential Assisted Living

National Association has experienced attorneys to help their members get passed these challenges.

The RAL National Association's mission is to provide the resources and support needed by RAL homeowners and operators. Avoiding obstacles as best you can, using other people's experience, knowledge and support is important. It is necessary as challenges arise with barriers created by cities, states, counties, homeowners' associations (HOAs), or others.

HOAs commonly exist in neighborhoods in newer and nicer communities. These associations ultimately have no legislative authority, they impose rules for the HOA members, and they cannot discriminate based on occupancy. HOAs do not have the power to override the Federal Fair Housing Act.

Even if they pay to retain a lawyer, ultimately, they will likely lose. With that in mind, we're not looking for a fight. We simply need to know the rules of the game and how to play by them. There are no federal rules regarding residential assisted living homes. Each state has its' own rules and guidelines. In a city or a local municipality, they do not have the power to undermine state laws and regulations.

Any law, rule, or regulation can be challenged and potentially reversed, changed, or waived.

The question you need to ask is, "Is it worth the effort?"

Let's use Dallas, Texas, as an example. The state allows 16 residents in a small RAL home, but the city of Dallas guidelines limit you to 8 seniors in homes within city limits. It's essential to know the rules of the game. The limit of 8 seniors can be challenged but ask yourself first if you are up to the fight. Having two homes with eight beds each would give you the same result without the hassle.

One way to work with rules like this is to establish a memory care-specific home instead of assisted living. Memory care homes typically have a lower census or number of residents.

They also charge higher rates. Knowing the existing rules and playing by them is essential. If you want to change the practices altogether, that's something different for the state or city where you work. Getting your home approved is your goal.

Changing a strategy within your business plan may help you overcome specific challenges. Adding a particular service, like memory care, may enable you to make more money. Other strategies include purchasing two homes nearby and hiring one team of employees that work at both. These strategies allow you to play by the rules and still win the game. In the state of Arizona, the maximum census is ten. I could battle that state regulation through legal court proceedings or continue to find ways to work within the system and win.

BUSINESS EXPENSES

There are expenses involved in owning and operating any business. Let's review the typical expenses for an average RAL home with ten beds. An average 10 bed RAL home could potentially produce gross income of $40,000 per month or more. This potential gross income is based on the national average cost of $4,300 per person for a private room according to Genworth, a long-term care insurance company.

The overhead expenses for a RAL business looks similar to a common household budget with a few additions.

Expenses include:
• Cable
• Internet
• Phone
• Newspaper
• Magazines
• Food
• Supplies
• Activities
• Landscaping
• Utilities
• Maintenance

The business of RAL also has additional expenses, such as:
• Staffing with caregivers and a manager
• Worker's compensation insurance for employees

- Marketing costs and fees paid to referral partners,
- Licensing and more.

BUILDING YOUR TEAM

THE KEY PLAYERS ON YOUR TEAM

1. Manager
2. Caregivers
3. Independent Contractors

We've discussed all the positions needed to operate an assisted living home effectively. Building your team is not just about hiring staff. You have to be prepared to train and retain them. Retention is essential in this industry. Most residential assisted living homeowners are familiar with the importance of maintaining a membership with the RAL National Association. One of the benefits of the organization is our online education for caregivers. Members of the Residential Assisted Living National Association can benefit from the additional education provided. In addition, your home can be included in our nationwide marketing map. You'll receive discounts with over 200 vendors, products and services, and gain access to the RALNA newsletter. The National Association provides the support needed to build your residential assisted living team and business along with legal advocacy and blogs.

STAFFING – EMPLOYEE OR INDEPENDENT CONTRACTOR?

You can pay your staff by the hour following the minimum wage and overtime rules in your state. If a state does not have a minimum wage requirement then you must follow the Federal minimum wage and overtime guidelines.

According to federal law, any salaried employee must still make at least the minimum wage plus time and a half for overtime.

The single largest expense for RAL is the staff. The staffing cost for an RAL home can be 40-50% or more of the gross income.

The combined expenses required to operate an assisted living home with ten residents can run $20,000 - $30,000 monthly or more, depending on many factors.

It's essential to calculate your income and expenses properly from the beginning. We created a tool called the Financial Suite, that we use to calculate the financial opportunity in an RAL business. The Financial Suite eliminates the guess work and shows what we can do to make the numbers work for us.

To learn more, go to www.RAL101.com

The great news is, a well-run RAL home can net 20-30% percent or more of the monthly gross income. With a $40,000 gross monthly income, that would potentially be $8,000 to $12,000 net per month.

It's important to note that caregivers should be classified and compensated as employees, not independent contractors.

As much as you may want to avoid having employees or attempt to call them independent contractors, they are not. This is very important so let me explain why that is.

Here is an easy way to determine if a caregiver SHOULD be classified as an employee or if they COULD be classified and compensated as an independent contractor.

- If they are scheduled regularly for a specific day and time, they are an employee. ICs can choose who they work for and what assignments they are willing to accept.
- If you do NOT allow them to work for someone else if they choose to, and you expect them to work solely or primarily for you, they are likely employees.

Are caregivers' employees or independent contractors?

1st - Caregivers in RAL homes DO have a schedule and they MUST be there to take care of the residents at the scheduled time. This is critical for the resident's care and well-being AND for the reputation of the business. They DO have a schedule so they are likely to be employees.

2nd - We would NOT want the caregivers to work for someone else and pick and choose between you and another employer. For those 2 reasons and many more, caregivers in RAL homes should be classified and compensated as employees.

On the other hand, if you ignore what you just learned and you decide to classify them as independent contractors anyway, there are some serious potential problems. Let me explain.

If your decision to classify them as independent contractors and not as employees is challenged and you cannot defend that decision, there are potential consequences.

1. You MAY have to pay their income taxes if they didn't pay them. That may not sound fair but that is the rule.
2. You MAY have to retroactively pay them the difference between what you did pay them and what you should have paid them if what you paid them didn't meet or exceed the minimum wage plus overtime requirements.
3. If you do have to pay them the difference retroactively, you MAY have to pay a penalty to the Department of Labor, of up to 100% of the amount you underpaid. Ouch!

It goes without saying, but we want to make sure we are doing this correctly. I've learned this from my own personal experience. When you follow our BLUEPRINT, you can avoid these mistakes.

Employee or IC, What's the Impact to my business?

Let me walk you through a common scenario that I've seen with people that are not aware of the rules or are choosing to not follow the rules I am sharing with you.

Keep in mind that, when you follow our BLUEPRINT, you can avoid many of these challenges and mistakes. We've already made many of these mistakes and we share them with you so that you can avoid making them yourself saving you money, time, and heartache.

A typical mom-and-pop RAL home may offer to pay caregivers as little as $3,000 as a monthly salary. That may come out to $150 a day for 5 days = $750 a week. They may pay them twice a month for a total of $3,000 a month. Conveniently skipping the 13th week each quarter. To sweeten the deal, they may offer them room and board in addition to the $3,000.

This would be a "live in" caregiver model and there are pros and cons that come with that model.

These caregivers are responsible for caring for the residents 24 hours a day, 5 days a week. The care home owner may call them independent contractors instead of employees to "save" them money. At least that's what they think will be the result.

The home owner is using the "live in" model. In their mind they may be justifying this because the caregiver is being paid a "salary" AND the caregiver is getting room and board in addition to the $3,000.

The thought is, the caregiver can take some breaks during the day, and they'll be able to sleep through most of the night. Thinking, maybe they'll only have to get up to help a resident a couple of times during the night. No big deal… or is it?

Keep in mind, the caregiver may be willing to accept that compensation especially if they are getting room and board as an additional part of their compensation. But that doesn't mean it follows the DOL's guidelines regarding minimum wage and overtime compensation.

3 POTENTIAL PROBLEMS WITH THE "LIVE IN" MODEL

First, the caregivers may not be getting paid enough to cover the required minimum wage plus overtime.

Second, the caregivers need a break to rest and recharge. Caregiving is not an easy job. It can be emotionally and physically demanding at times. And the caregiver may even have a family and kids of their own that need their attention.

Third, since part of their compensation is housing, they are essentially a tenant of the business. If you decide you no longer want to continue to employ that caregiver, you can terminate their employment.

But now you have the challenge of removing them as a tenant. The rules and regulations for evicting a tenant can be complicated. Imagine being stuck with a disgruntled tenant living inside your RAL home. That could be a recipe for some serious problems as well. It's important to mention again that your residents ARE NOT tenants. The residents are receiving a service that you are providing. That is the "care" we provide. That isn't the same as a tenant landlord relationship.

Let me illustrate what you would be required to pay a caregiver in compensation if they are a live-in caregiver and they are required to be responsible 24 hours a day for 5 days a week at a $10 per hour minimum wage.

Keep in mind we still need to staff the home during the other 2 days a week. To simplify this example, I am leaving out the "other" 2 days a week and any taxes or workmen's compensation insurance.

24 hours X 5 days = 120 hours a week.
The 1st 40 hours are compensated at $10 per hour = $400
The 80 overtime hours are at $15 per hour = $1,200.
The total compensation for those 5 days would be $1,600.
With 4.3 weeks per month that would be $6,880.

There is a HUGE difference between the $3,000 "salary" they may be willing to accept and the $6,880 you could be "required" to pay them.

You can put a "reasonable" dollar value for the room and board you are providing and include that as a part of their compensation. But $3,880 is probably not going to be considered "reasonable." Even if you said the room and board had a value of $1,000 a month, that is still a huge difference.

If you do provide the room and board as a part of the compensation, the caregiver would be required to pay the income taxes on that value as if it were cash compensation.

YOU may like that, but the caregiver will not. So now you are wondering, "what can I do?" Let me give you some alternatives that would be better for you and the caregiver.

First, Give the Caregiver a break!

Being a caregiver is a stressful career. They will need to have a break to rest and recharge. Let's make sure they do have adequate opportunity to rest and recharge. **And let's also avoid paying overtime as much as we can.**

If they do get 8 hours "off duty" during the day and they are not responsible to take care of residents during those 8 hours, it would be a 16 hour shift per day for the caregiver.

Here's what the "16 hour shift" model looks like

16 hours X 5 Days = 80 hours.
That's less hours of overtime BUT we still need to hire another caregiver to cover those remaining 8 hours each day.

40 hours X $10 per hour = $400.
40 hours X $15 per hour = $600. Overtime at time and a half.

(Assuming another caregiver covers the remaining 40 hours)
40 hours X $10 per hour = $400.
The total is, $400 + $600 + $400 = $1,400
That's a savings of $200 a week.

$1,400 X 4.3 weeks per month = $6,020
That's a total $860 total saved per month.
Better but not the best.

A better way to compensate the caregiving staff without having to pay excessive over time might look like this.

1. Use 12 hour shifts vs 24 hour or 16 hour shifts.
2. Limit your staff to 3 shifts a week for a total of 36 hours. That eliminates overtime compensation completely. Some caregivers will want more hours or more shifts.

Now you have a choice:
You can decide to allow them to take on overtime hours knowing you'll be paying a higher pay rate if you do.

If you have more than 1 home, that is not under common ownership, that can help. Or you can "share" your staff with another care home so that both of you avoid paying overtime. IE: each home hires a caregiver for 2 or 3 shifts.

3. Even though shorter shifts require additional staff, it also creates some added benefits.
   ○ You can reduce the cost of overtime.

- You're giving the caregiver time to rest & recharge
- They can be available for extra shifts as needed.

Here is what that looks like financially when you can eliminate overtime completely.
24 hours X $10 per hour = $240 a day X 5 days = $1,200
$1,200 X 4.3 weeks each month = $5,160.

The "live in" model cost is potentially $6,680 per month
The "16 + 8 hour" shift model is potentially $6,020
The "no overtime" model is potentially $5,160 a month.

What does the full cost of the labor look like?
Let's assume we used the "no overtime" model.
We also need to cover the "other" 2 days each week.
2 days X 24 hours X $10 per hour = $480 a week
X 4.3 weeks = $2,064.

You are required to provide 24 hour care 7 days a week.
1st 5 days = $5,160 + the "other" 2 days at $2,064 = $7,224.
In addition, there will be taxes and workmen's compensation insurance on top of that.

BLUEPRINT suggest that you have a caregiver ratio of 5 or 6 residents to 1 caregiver during that day and 1 care giver at night for 10 or 12 residents.

To reach the caregiver to resident ratio needed during the day we would need to add a 2nd caregiver. Using the "no overtime" method we would add $3,612 per month

12 hours a day X 7 days = 84 hours X $10 per hour = $840 a week X 4.3 weeks per month = $3,612 per month.

$7,224 + $3,612 = $10,836
Rounding that up to cover the taxes and insurance that would be about $12,500 per month.

What does the compensation for a manager look like?

First of all, it is not a full-time job to manage 1 RAL home. A good manager can manage 2, 3, 4 or more RAL homes. If they manage 3 or 4 homes at $1,500 per month they can earn $4,500 - $6,000 or more.

MANAGERS CAN BE INDEPENDENT CONTRACTORS FOR 2 REASONS.

1. They can choose to manage more than 1 home
2. They do not have a "set" schedule.

A caregiver can be a manager and a caregiver.

If you have a caregiver that is also acting as your manager they can be compensated with a higher hourly rate, a flat monthly rate or they can be paid by the hour for any "manager" duties.

If we add $1,500 a month for a manager, the total staffing costs would be about $14,000 or so per month. With some occasional overtime or last minute replacement shifts lets round that up to $15,000 a month. As you can see, the staffing cost is the largest single category of all.

The BLUPRINT formula suggests the staffing costs should be no more than 40-50% of the gross income to have a very profitable RAL business. $40,000 X 40% = $16,000. That is the BLUPRINT formula for success in the RAL business.

THE RAL BUSINESS BLUEPRINT

According to the National Center for Assisted Living (NCAL), there are about 30,000 assisted living communities in America today. About 65% have 21 beds or less and the rest, typically, have 100 beds or more. The homes with 21 beds or less are what we call, RAL homes. They are typically residential homes in a neighborhood with no sign in front. 100 beds or more are what we call "Big Box" Assisted Living communities.

Many of the RAL homes existing today are "mom-and-pop" operations. They are typically owned and operated by somebody who lives in the house and they provide the care for the residents themselves. They have few if any employees and they have little if any freedom of time.

In reality, they don't own a business, it owns them...

They are the manager, caregiver, cook, baker, and the candlestick maker. This is NOT the BLUEPRINT formula.

The BLUEPRINT formula starts with a beautiful home in a great neighborhood located in the proper location. You hire a manager, and they choose the caregivers. Do it once and then repeat the process to create as many homes as you desire.

HOW SHOULD I STRUCTURE
THE BUSINESS ENTITIES?

I'm not an attorney, and I'm not giving you legal advice. I will share what I do, and you can decide what's best for you. Choosing the proper structure is very important and it helps with asset protection and provides flexibility.

I own the real estate in one entity, and I operate the business in a separate entity. You can lease the real estate from your own entity that owns it. You can pay your own entity the rent and you can choose the amount that you will charge yourself too.

The higher the rent your real estate entity charges your assisted living entity, the more you will be able to write off in business deductions. That higher income can be offset by the accelerated depreciation strategies available on the real estate. The BLUPRINT provides the best business model for RALs across the country for individuals who want to do good and do well. We found and vetted, asset protection and tax experts to teach students more about the potential entity structures during our 3-day fast track training.

BLUEPRINT is intended to give you an overview of all the components involved in Residential Assisted Living. The RAL Academy's 3 day FAST TRACK Immersion training goes into more detail on this important topic.

The actual entities can be LLCs, C-Corps, sole proprietors or more. It is always best to work with Asset protection and tax professionals to determine the best entity formation for you. If you would like to learn more about who we use for our legal and accounting needs, Check out the RAL National Association at www.RALNA.org.

Many of the companies that we work with are also a part of our "partner network" at the RALNA. You'll find a list of these partners at the RALNA website.

HANDS-ON OR HANDS-OFF?

If you want to be a "hands off" owner or Operator of a RAL home, it may be better for you to select a location that is farther away. The closer the home is to you, the more likely you may be tempted to stop in and get involved and eventually you will be "hands on." I say keep your hands to yourself...

In the BLUEPRINT formula, your primary role as the owner is to manage the manager. Empowering your manager to be successful is your primary focus. They need guidelines, goals, and resources to be successful. Your role is to make sure the business is profitable and runs smoothly. Your function is to make sure the money comes in, and the money goes out. It would be wise to perform spot checks on your business from time to time.

However, you should invest your time working "on" your business and not "in" your business. Successful owners should focus on the "Big" picture and not get sucked into the daily operations of the company.

SHOULD I DO IT IN MY OWN BACKYARD?

Don't limit yourself to only owning a RAL home near your personal home. This could be a recipe for "over-involvement."

Hire the right people, put them in the correct positions, give them the authority and provide them with the tools and resources they need. Then stand back and be prepared to offer support when necessary.

When your business operates like a well-oiled machine in your absence, that's when you know you own the company, and it doesn't own you. When your staff makes decisions that you disagree with, consider that a training opportunity and offer suggestions and more options for the future. Otherwise, you'll find yourself in a position where your business owns you instead of you owning the business. Embrace the idea of making money without having to be on sight every day. That may require you to change the way you've been thinking.

AVOID THE MEDICARE/ MEDICAID MODEL

Elderly residents that are relying on Medicare and Medicaid typically have $3,000 or less available per month to pay for their care. That may be a combination of social security and a supplement from the state.

Most individuals who are NOT relying on the government to provide their care are paying in the range of $3,000 to $8,000 monthly. And some pay even more.

We call these residents "private pay" residents. The BLUE-PRINT formula focuses on "private pay" residents. The fact is, you have a limited number of beds and you have a choice as to who you serve. In order to "Do Good And Do Well" we focus on the higher paying residents. This allows us to provide a better experience overall.

If I can afford a nicer home in a better area and I can pay caregivers more, attracting the best caregivers, and provide better food, entertainment, and amenities...

That results in a better experience overall. That is one of the keys to the BLUEPRINT formula.

Medicare and Medicaid are federal government programs that provide funding to the state. In turn, the state creates a program that typically pays $2,000 or less a month for assisted living, including all the resident's sources of income.

RAL homeowners who accept these low rates may not be able to make a reasonable profit. Or they may not be able to provide high quality care in a safe area that our BLUEPRINT formula calls for.

RAL homes that focus on residents subsidized by the government, may only bring in $20,000 a month in gross income. After expenses are paid, the business may be unable to survive. That type of a scenario is more of a "labor of love" or it may even be a charity. That is not what we are looking to do using the BLUEPRINT formula.

This is why our BLUEPRINT encourages owners to offer nicer homes in better areas so we can charge higher rates of $4,000-$8,000 or more per month.

BLUEPRINT is not solely based on what we charge; it's also the location, level of care required, amenities, quality of caregivers, and other services we offer.

If the average today is $4,300 per person per month, what if we were able to charge $5,000 instead?

How would this help you and your residents?

At $5,000 per person, with ten residents, you are now potentially grossing $50,000 monthly. That extra $10,000 enables you to potentially hire even better caregivers and pay them even more. You could provide better food and entertainment, and perhaps a culinary-trained chef.

Now think even bigger and imagine having 16 residents in your home at $5,000 per month or more…

1. How big of a home could you provide?
2. How nice of an area could it be in?
3. What amenities & entertainment could you offer?
4. How much more money could you make?

While we place a lot of emphasis on location, there are five keys to owning and operating a profitable residential assisted living home.

THE 5 KEYS TO SUCCESS IN RAL

"There are five keys to success that every RAL owner and operator should know and use to help ensure their success and accelerate their start-up phase."

THE FIVE KEYS TO SUCCESS

In the RAL BLUEPRINT formula there are five keys to success that we teach our students.

1. Location
2. Team
3. Clients
4. Getting Paid
5. Systems

KEY #1: CHOOSING THE RIGHT LOCATION

When I first started building my RAL business, there was no proven process or step by step guide to follow. I analyzed the market, the competition and the opportunity and then I created and perfected the BLUEPRINT formula you are learning right now.

3 CRITICAL ELEMENTS WHEN SELECTING THE BEST LOCATION:

1. The demographics & financial strength of the community.
2. The physical convenience to access the home.
3. The competition today and the competition that's coming.

WHO IS REALLY YOUR CLIENT?

To better understand "where" we should have our RAL home we need to better define "WHO" we are really looking for.

Keep in mind, the target demographic you are looking for is not the actual residents in your home, it's their children.

Your target client is the resident's children.
Those 50-60 year old "children" will be the ones choosing the location. And they will also be responsible for paying for their parent's housing and care.

Important characteristics of the target demographic:

1. **Homeowners vs. renters.** This indicates stability and a higher income or access to financial resources.
2. **Higher average age group.** We target 50–60-year-olds because their parents will typically be 80-90 years old.
3. **Twice the average household income** in the immediate geographic area. By targeting higher income areas, you will likely be locating people with the ability to pay higher rates. And those people will want to have

better than average homes for their parents and they will have the ability to pay for that housing and care.

THE 5 LEVELS OF RAL HOMES

The BLUEPRINT formula identifies 5 levels based on:
1. Location and convenience in getting to the home
2. Quality of the home and the surrounding neighborhood
3. Demographics and the financial ability to pay higher than average rates for their parent's housing and care.

Level 1 homes are typically in questionable neighborhoods that you wouldn't want to slow your car down in, let alone have your mom or dad live there. These homes get the lowest rates and provide below average amenities and care

Level 5 targets the nicest homes in the best locations. The reality is many times the real estate is more expensive than is needed to maximize the profit of the RAL business. These homes command the highest rates.

Level 3 and level 4 Homes are the Sweet Spot
Level 3 or 4 homes give us the best combination of location, demographics, affordability, and profit potential.

The location of your RAL home can make or break your business. "Over the river and through the woods to Grandmother's house we go" are lyrics we sing during the holidays. In reality, we want it to be close and to be very convenient when visiting loved ones in a RAL home.

The location also plays a factor in maximizing or limiting your profit potential. The location also plays a factor when it comes to hiring and retaining employees.

I cannot emphasize this enough; the **Location is key.**

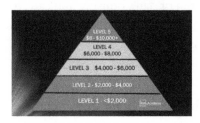

Level 3 or level 4 RAL homes are above the middle but not at the very top. The price range per person is typically in the $4,000 to $8,000 range. The rates they pay will depend on the location, the level of care provided and the amenities and services that you provide.

Prices will vary just like they do in a restaurant.

You can pay $20 for a steak dinner, or you can pay $200 for a steak dinner. There are many variables determining the price someone is willing to pay for it.

A high-end revolving roof top restaurant in a downtown skyscraper is going to command a higher price for that steak than a run-down shack inconveniently located in the middle of nowhere.

The same holds true for Residential Assisted Living.

Keep in mind that some people are happy and even proud to tell their friends how much they paid for things. That could be either the $20 or the $200. When it comes to paying for mom or dad's housing and care, for some, there is no limit. They will pay for the best of the best. It may seem odd to you, but they may even *WANT* to pay the highest rates possible.

This could be for many reasons including:
1. They have the means to pay more, and they want to provide "the best" of everything for their parents.
2. They believe they will be getting better care or better services and amenities if they are paying a higher rate
3. They may be feeling "guilty" and paying higher rates may help them to cope with that guilt.

The BLUEPRINT formula focuses on clients that have the financial ability to choose the level of home they live in. These are typically "private pay" clients, and they can afford to pay higher rates than the "average" person can afford to pay.

We select the most appropriate homes in the best locations and we use the BLUEPRINT formula to maximize our profits.

Not every senior who needs housing and care can afford to pay for it on their own. They may ultimately be subsidized by the government or even a fraternal organization they belong to.

The BLUEPRINT formula is focused on "private pay" clients, not on government-assisted or otherwise subsidized clients.

BIGGER IS BETTER WHEN IT COMES TO THE SQUARE FOOTAGE OF THE HOME ITSELF

When it comes to the size of the home itself, the bigger the better... But don't go overboard.

The BLUEPRINT formula says that 300 square feet per person or more is suitable for a very comfortable RAL home. That means that a 3,000 sf home could house 10 or 12 residents comfortably.

According to most state guidelines, you can use a 1,800 square foot home and house ten residents. That is not very comfortable in my opinion, and that is not what we encourage.

The number of bedrooms and bathrooms can be increased or decreased within the square footage of the home.

Even though you can have 2 people in each bedroom, you'll want as many private bedrooms as possible. A combination of private and semi-private bedrooms is common.

You will need a minimum of 2 full or ¾ bathrooms as well. Providing private bedrooms and bathrooms allows you to charge the residents a higher rate. You will not find many 10 bed 10 bath homes on the market. Creatively using the space you have or strategically adding space will allow you to maximize the number of bedrooms and bathrooms in your RAL home.

Bathrooms are more challenging to add than converting space into more bedrooms. In almost every state, the minimum you'll need is two bathrooms. The more bathrooms, the better. You will typically charge more for private bathrooms. **More square footage will provide you with space to better accommodate the residents in your RAL home.**

You may be thinking "small" right now. You may even be thinking to yourself "I'm going to start small to get started. I'll start with a 3 bedroom house and have two people per room to get started." If that is what you are thinking, hear me clearly, **That would be a mistake my friend.**

Here's why. It's just as much effort to start a "small" and potentially much less profitable, home than it is to start with a larger and potentially, much more profitable home.

Adding bathrooms will provide a better experience and allow you to charge more if they are private bathrooms. Bedrooms are easier to add than the plumbing required for a bathroom. Regardless, compare the cost and the income it will generate. If you spend $5,000 to add a bathroom and you can charge $500 a month more, it will pay for itself in less than 1 year. That is a high value improvement that is well worth the cost.

Larger homes are likely to cost more money. Compare a 3,000 square foot house with a 4,800 square feet home. With 1,800 additional square feet, allotting 300 square feet per resident, that allows room for six more residents potentially.

Even better, instead of charging $3,000 or $4,000 monthly in a less expensive home, you may be able to charge $5,000 to $6,000 in a bigger and nicer home. The larger home may have space for 16 seniors, each paying $5000 per month, versus ten people paying $3,000. **This is why you shouldn't settle for the "minimum" when you are getting started. I want to encourage you to follow the step by step BLUEPRINT formula. Think bigger, and scale.** If you do choose to use a larger home, it should more than pay for itself.

To help make the best decision, use these 3 questions to help evaluate the opportunity
1. What's the total investment in time, effort & money?
2. What is the gross and net income potential?
3. What's the return on my investment of time & money?

Whenever you think of starting small, think again. Too many potential business owners have the minimalist mindset of starting small before learning the process. Now, with the RAL BLUEPRINT formula you can clearly see that for yourself.

ZONING AND HOAS

Understanding the "rules of the game" is important. We want you to understand how zoning and HOAs work. Sometimes state rules and municipal regulations can be convoluted and cumbersome. This is why we urge owners and operators to join the Residential Assisted Living National Association (www.RALNA.com).

The association has a legal team that is experienced in avoiding delays and stumbling blocks that can delay your start-up process. Some states have a host of licensing requirements, and others have much less, you should consider taking extra precautions to keep seniors safe regardless.

In summary, choosing the right location is critical to the success of your RAL home. The sweet spot is level 3 or level 4 homes.

The goal of the RAL Academy's 3-Day FAST TRACK Immersion class, is to provide in-depth training on every area you'll need to be start, own, operate or invest in a RAL home.

To learn more about the RAL 3 Day FAST TRACK Immersion class, go to: www.RAL101.com

SUCCESS KEY #2.
TEAM, MAKING PEOPLE A PRIORITY

Unquestionably, residential assisted living is about making people your priority. This business is centered on taking care of people. If you are willing to take special care of your staff, they will be more likely to provide the same level of care to the residents.

If your goal is to make money, you will first have to learn how to make residents your priority. The care you provide to the residents is a critical component of your business, superseding real estate.

For potential business owners and investors who are thinking, "I'm all about the money, I don't care about people," this business is not for you until you change your philosophy.

For me the change in my purpose for even doing RAL changed from being a business opportunity to providing great care when it was my mother who needed the help.

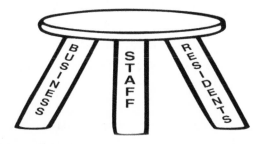

SUCCESS KEY #3. CLIENTS AND RESIDENTS

Think of your business as a three-legged stool with three separate but equal legs.

1. The Business
2. The Residents
3. The Staff

If you make the mistake of overlooking one leg of your stool, it will fall. Remember, when considering the three-legged stool, each leg is equally important. If you don't care about people, this is the wrong business for you. If you don't see the value of operating a profitable business and don't care about making money, this is the wrong Blueprint. You have to keep your heart, motives, and wallet in balance. Your residents, the staff, and the business are equally important. When you keep all three legs balanced, your business will soar. This type of balance is what "Doing Good and Doing Well" is all about.

SUCCESS KEY #4. GETTING PAID

Getting paid is the key to success for any profitable business. As mentioned previously, our residential assisted living Blueprint does not focus on Medicare and Medicaid. Veterans that are eligible for VA benefits can receive a few thousand dollars a month. These funds can be used for assisted living, and their own money can supplement that too.

We focus on residents that are private pay or have Long Term Care Insurance. Ultimately, it is the families' responsibility to take care of this payment, regardless of the source of money.

SUCCESS KEY #5.
PUTTING SYSTEMS IN PLACE

The final key to success is systems. You, and your manager, must have proven systems in place for everything to operate smoothly.

Systems include:
1. real estate,
2. renovations,
3. your team,
4. policies and procedures,
5. funding, and business partners.

Attending the Residential Assisted Living Academy allows individuals to understand better how these systems should be put in place. Visit: www.RALAcademy.com to learn how to execute your plans.

THE REAL ESTATE

There must be systems built around the real estate we use for operating the business with residential assisted living. You need to know where to locate the home, fund it, and acquire it. In addition to location, you may need to raise capital. Raising capital for residential assisted living is one of the easier things I've ever raised capital for, but I've been doing it for 40 years.

At the RAL Academy training, we spend time teaching you the formulas, the secrets and the skills that we've discovered over the years.

To raise capital, you will need to articulate your business plan in words and writing. At the RAL Academy 3-Day FAST TRACK Immersion class, we teach students the elements of a successful business plan, the best ways to fund the acquisition and the renovation of the real estate, and funding for the business start-up as well.

RENOVATIONS

When making renovations, you will need to know what to do and what not to do. I love visiting people's RAL homes across the country, whether they're students of the academy or not.

During one visit to a non-student's RAL home, I remember complimenting the home's beauty.

As they explained all the renovations they made, I was adding up the cost in my mind. They completed about $80,000 to $100,000 worth of renovations that they could have avoided.

They experienced so many missed steps and losses that it was sad to know that those mistakes could have been avoided.

Instead of going through the RALA 3-day training or even completing the home study course, they decided to try to figure it out by themselves.

They did it, but it cost them over $80,000 more money out of pocket. That's a substantial and unnecessary loss. By investing a few thousand into their education, they would have completed their home in a lot less time for a lot less money and they would have made more money, faster.

POLICIES AND PROCEDURES

All RAL homes must have policies and procedures in writing and approved. Unfortunately, the state agencies do not issue policies and procedures to follow.

You provide the state with your proposed policies and guidelines on how you plan to operate the home.

In return, they inform you if your plans are acceptable. Here's the catch, whatever you say you're going to do, the state will hold you accountable for it.

My initial policies and procedures were in a binder that was about 3 inches thick. I was proud. I had mimicked the policies of a popular "Big Box" facility. I didn't know any better because I had no one to teach me.

During my initial inspection, I felt prepared, but I wasn't. The surveyor explained that I had many guidelines and rules in my policies and procedures that I didn't need.

She couldn't go into detail about the revisions required. Well thanks a lot! I ultimately did figure it out but that delay alone delayed me from opening the home for 30 days.

That means I had no income for those 30 days.

That is a huge financial hit to the bottom line.

However, since then, my policy and procedures consist of need-to-know information like emergency plans, balanced meals, and other critical components. When you have good managers, they will make sure the policy and procedures you've designed are carried out. When you attend the RAL Academy 3-day FAST TRACK Immersion class, you can see the same policies and procedures that I use.

FUNDING

The golden question for every new business owner is, "How do I get funding for this?" It's a residential property. You can do any type of non-owner-occupied residential loan. The bank only has to know that it's a non-owner-occupied home loan - this implies that the buyer is planning to lease the property. You can even have a signed lease with the entity that will be renting the house from you. A 5-year lease at a high rate will be comforting to a potential lender. As a result, lenders may allow you to negotiate an even higher loan or better terms, if necessary. These are the kind of professional tips students learn at the RAL academy. Knowledge makes the business process flow smoothly. Otherwise, individuals are left to figure it all out on their own.

BUSINESS PARTNERS

If you need a partner, get one. However, if you can hire someone to do the job you are looking for them to do, then reconsider the need to partner. Sometimes, you hear people say, "I'll never do business with friends and family." So, what's the alternative, enemies or strangers? Think about it, if we become friends while owning a business together, do we need to dissolve the company? Of course not. We have to change our logic about business. I do business with family all the time. It doesn't matter if it's a family business. You still need to discuss and decide on the details upfront. Be sure to ask a series of questions before partnering in business – this will save you a lot of heartaches, disappointment, and loss.

WORK ON YOUR BUSINESS, NOT IN YOUR BUSINESS

I've read that Sir Richard Branson has nearly 400 companies, and not one has a personal office. He doesn't micromanage. He creates the company, puts the right person in charge, and provides the needed tools and resources. It's okay to visit your business and make yourself available as needed. More importantly, put the right person in charge, and your responsibilities will diminish drastically - this is how I keep traveling and working on my business, because I'm not working in my industry – I'm able to live my life freely. You have to decide on how you want to live your life as a business owner.

My manager and my caregivers allow me to live my life and continue working on my business. The manager and the caregivers are probably the most important people in my assisted living organization. The manager and my caregivers are face-to-face with residents day-to-day. More importantly, they are face-to-face with the family members. Family members see added value when caregivers share a loving relationship with their mothers and fathers.

Significant decisions are marked by broadening your perspective as a business owner. Success demands that you take action. What actions are you taking to establish a successful residential assisted living business today?

Far too many business owners work in their companies and not on them. As a result, they fail to flourish. If you are looking for a speedy entry into the industry, immediately contact the RAL academy to join the next training.

DOES THE RAL BUSINESS HAVE VALUE BY ITSELF?

Yes it does. Let me share a case study to illustrate the potential value of the business alone. For example, we helped one student negotiate a $275,000 asking price down to $230,000. The real estate was worth $180,000, and the business was purchased for just $50,000. This student used the BLUEPRINT formula, implemented better business practices, transitioned higher-paying residents into the home, reselling it for a significant profit.

The real estate was still valued at $180,000 and was sold for that. The business sold for $150,000 for a combined price of $330,000. She made a profit of $100,000 in less than 1 year.

This is one way your assisted living business can grow fast. The business was purchased at $50,000 initially, and then sold for $150,000. That was because of the increased cash flow. A business is worth what somebody is willing to pay for it. The increased cash flow of the business increased its value by 3X.

The RAL business valuation is based on two primary factors:
1. The cash flow.
2. The potential for the future.

OPERATING PROCEDURES

*"Finding quality staff and filling your home
with high paying clients are two of the most
important operating procedures RAL business
owners need to learn."*

PAYING EMPLOYEES

Caregivers are some of the most important players, yet
they are also paid the least. They usually earn a few dollars
over minimum wage. For example, if your state's minimum
wage is $10, they are likely to make $10 to $13 an hour.
In Arizona, the minimum wage increased from $8.05 an
hour to $12 over the course of the past few years

I've never paid employees $8.05.

We started caregivers off at $9 years ago. After they're employed
for a length of time, we increased their pay to $10. Upon two
years of employment, our caregivers earned about $11 an hour.
Now, our pay scale has been forced to change for everyone.

What happens when the minimum wage goes up? A new
employee starts by earning the same $12 an hour that
another caregiver had to work years to get.

That long standing caregiver will likely request a wage increase, and rightfully so. Unfortunately, this is the perspective the government fails to calculate when interfering with minimum wage laws. Elected officials will argue that only 3 percent of the population earns minimum wage. This argument fails because increasing the minimum wage affects more than just the 3 percent. So, guess what happens next? As a result, all our assisted living residents receive an increase in their monthly fees to cover the added expenses of paying employees a higher rate.

Businesses will pass on the additional cost, or they will have to cut back on the quality of the care. Cutting back isn't an option with the Blueprint, so the increase is passed along.

FINDING QUALITY CAREGIVERS

When you visit our assisted living homes and meet our caregivers, it looks like the United Nations. Our caregivers come in all shapes, sizes, and genders from all over the world. They come from Romania, the Philippines, Russia, North Africa, Mexico, and the United States.

To find the best caregivers, no matter where they are from, we use specific criteria to communicate expectations and to secure, qualified caregivers. It's essential to create a team that is not all about the money, genuinely loves seniors, and does a good job caring for their needs.

COOKS, CAREGIVERS, AND CHEFS

While the house manager makes sure food is in the home, caregiver duties often require food preparation skills. If you have a higher-level home, the meal preparation can be done by a professionally trained culinary chef. These chefs add an ambiance with their traditional white jackets and white hats. They provide cooked-to-order breakfast and lunch. Between breakfast and lunch, they prepare the dinner that the caregivers will serve during the evening shift.

With the rise of TV shows on the Cooking Channel and the Food Network, an influx of inspired individuals eagerly registered for culinary school.

Upon graduation, they cannot find jobs, but they have a passion for putting their culinary art on display. Sometimes, it's easier to hire chefs than caregivers. It allows them the opportunity and experience to show off their skills and obtain a sense of satisfaction cooking for a home occupied by ten appreciative residents. These chefs usually work for the same pay as caregivers, and depending on their culinary talents, they may be paid a little more.

UNIQUE SERVICES

In addition to managers, caregivers, and chefs, assisted living homes may require additional independent contractors' unique services from time to time. Independent contractors can include hairstylists, people who conduct yoga classes for seniors, musicians for entertainment, pet therapy, and even a handyman. Our manager has a list of contractors we routinely use for tradespeople who work on the roof, plumbing, electrical and more. They resolve the issue, and I typically find out about it when the bill comes.

If it's a larger expense, maybe a decision to repair or replace a water heater, I get an advance call. If I'm unavailable or can't be reached, my manager has the authority to make the decision. Upon my return, I either say, "Job well done," or I'll explain what I would have done differently. Ultimately, I allow my staff space and opportunity to do the best job possible. Supporting and empowering them in this way creates a team that knows what to do and one that can operate efficiently.

IDENTIFYING THE CLIENTS

Who are the clients? Contrary to what most people think, our clients are not the residents in the home. Our clients are typically the adult children of the residents who live in the house. During our RAL 3-Day FAST TRACK Immersion class, we use an avatar we've named "Daughter Judy." This is the designated person appointed as the family's spokesperson. It is the "Daughter Judy" of every family that we ultimately have to keep satisfied - this is usually the one person responsible for making the decisions for the loved ones. Ultimately, they are responsible for paying for the care the residents receive.

A fall at a resident's own home frequently leads to mom or dad moving into a RAL home. If "Daughter Judy" communicates that the family is placing a parent in the house so that they will "never fall again," a conversation is needed. Being in an assisted living home does not eliminate fall risks. However, we can be there in the event of a fall, and we know exactly how to respond. If there is a severe issue, we call 911 for immediate emergency response. The overall health of a resident will not miraculously improve because they moved into an assisted living, but we provide the best care possible. As trained professionals, we take the highest precautions and provide professional care, but sometimes things happen - this is why I recommend professional business liability insurance for residential assisted living homes. That insurance costs less than you might think since we do not provide medical services.

A GOOD IN-TAKE ASSESSMENT

Keep in mind that assisted living homes are not obligated to accept any residents – we are not landlords – we provide a service. Assisted living in-take standards are subjective. As a result, owners can say "no" and reject a resident based on any criteria whatsoever, even if "Daughter Judy" is too demanding or unreasonable. During our 3-day fast track training, we share insights with our students on how to do proper intake assessments to save time and money in the future. These assessments should always be done face-to-face. We avoid many difficult situations because we conduct detailed assessments to avert potential problems as much as possible. It's sporadic, but they can be removed from the home if a resident fails to pay. They are not tenants, and we are not landlords. We provide a service. If we can't offer the assistance, they need or cannot pay for the service we provide, the resident will have to move out of the home.

WHAT HAPPENS IF THE RESIDENT CAN'T PAY?

When financial problems occur, we still function as a friendly business – we have a heart. Remember, people, matter to our business. If they are running out of money, "Daughter Judy" will likely call to explain that they only have $10,000 remaining, and their monthly fee is $5,000. What should you do in difficult situations like this? You have options. You can instruct the family to apply for state Medicaid or Medicare benefits. Once the family applies with proof of limited income and assets, they may qualify for a supplement that may add up to about $2,000 per month. This amount includes their pension, if any, and their social security. That would leave a balance of $3,000 that needs to be paid. Moving mom into a shared room may offset the expenses by $1,000, and the family could pay the difference. If not, we would help them move their mom to another assisted living home.

There was a scenario when I purchased an existing residential assisted living business, and one resident had been there for almost ten years. Her point of contact was a distant niece who lived on the other side of the country – she visited twice a year. The niece called and explained that her great aunt's money was running out, and they could not pay for it themselves. I instructed her to apply for the state benefits. I let them know that I would accept whatever the state would pay – allowing her to stay for the rest of her life. She'd already been there for nine-plus years. In this case, I decided to go without a couple of thousand dollars a month. I didn't want her to go someplace else for the last few months of her life. That is a part of being able to "Do Good and Do Well."

Waiving or reducing fees should be a rare option. Adjusting what residents pay based on family members cannot create an unwanted reputation for your business. People will quickly realize that you are willing to accept less than you should. They might even intentionally pay you $5,000 for a few months and then transition to state benefits to stay in your mid-level home with waived fees. Even worse, they could cause you to go out of business – remember the 3-legged stool. Family members are ultimately your clients, not the potential residents living in your home.

DEATH BENEFITS CAN BE SOLD

Did you know that you can sell the future death benefits of your life insurance policy for cash today? The owner can sell the death benefit while the insured is still alive. The older the insured, the greater the present value of that future death benefit. Life insurance is primarily used to replace your income for your living dependents after you pass away. When someone is between 60-80 years of age, their children are usually independent adults, no longer in need of supplemental income. If they cancel the policy to save money on the premium or withdraw the policy's cash value, they will do themselves a dreadful disservice. If they don't need the future death benefit, selling the death benefit may best serve seniors. As a result, a policy could be worth 40-50 cents on the dollar, based on the insured's age.

You might be wondering why a company would pay for the death benefit of a policy? They use an algorithm to calculate the amount they are willing to pay using the age and health of the insured to determine the current value of the policy. Based on all of that, they factor the buyout of the death benefits at a rate of return they are willing to accept. Learn more at: https://www.harborlifesettlements.com.

Most people aren't familiar with this process. Decisions to cancel and cash in a policy are made when adult children are unaware of their insurance options and cannot pay the premiums. As a result, they withdraw the insurance policy's cash value and stop paying the premiums, giving up the future death benefit entirely. Sometimes, the logic behind this strategy is to qualify for Long-Term care benefits. Unfortunately, there is a 5-year "look back" rule when the state reviews the estate's value over the previous five years; the claim for benefits may be denied. Instead, they could have potentially sold the insurance for hundreds of thousands of dollars, and this would have provided the funds to pay for assisted living needs. After that, they could apply and qualify for state benefits. Use this information to help new clients transition their parents into senior care without making uneducated and harmful decisions. These professional tips help ensure that you can inform clients and make sure that you will get paid.

LONG TERM CARE INSURANCE

Another highly reliable source to ensure that you get paid is long-term care insurance. When clients communicate that mom or dad has long-term care insurance, it's like listening to angels sing. Typically, these individuals purchased long-term care policies more than 30-years-ago. These benefits may have started by providing $100 a day for assisted living care. For policies written years ago, there is typically no waiting period to transition into the home. The rate of $100 per day doesn't sound like enough to cover the expenses for our residential assisted living model. However, the policies usually allot for a 3-4 percent annual cost-of-living increase. The $100 per day may have increased to $300 a day, based on the age of the policy. Some students immediately reply, "But Gene, what if you're only charging $4,000 for the room? How would that cost-of-living increase help?" Here is the good part - this is why your agreement with the residents should indicate that you will charge the "maximum allowable" amount in such cases.

In most cases that involve long-term care insurance, it's to your benefit to bill the highest amount possible. If you do not do this, the insurance company will keep the money. To avoid this from happening, read every policy thoroughly. I've encountered people who have been in the business for 16 years that were not aware of this Long-Term Care insurance strategy.

CREATING A COMMUNITY

*"Sales cure cash flow problems in businesses,
and all sales start with marketing."*

MARKETING YOUR
ASSISTED LIVING HOME

Make sure you are marketing to the right people. Maintaining the proper marketing perspective will enable you to land potential clients. Some essential marketing tools are proven to work:

- Websites
- Flyers
- Brochures
- Business Cards
- Social Media Pages

In addition to the basics, if you can display a sign in front of the home, do so. However, most residential neighborhoods will not permit you to display a commercial sign. Do not allow residential restrictions to hinder your marketing efforts – be creative. For example, when communities restrict signage, perhaps try using big bright letters on the mailbox. Then again, maybe it's not a sign at all; consider using lawn decoration within the landscaping. Considering that residential assisted living homes are located within residential neighborhoods, hosting open houses is effective and inexpensive. Invite your surrounding neighbors, but only after you've opened your home.

MARKETING TO HOAS

More than likely, there will be some form of opposition coming from some neighbors. When you are getting started, complete your necessary paperwork, do your renovations, plan for your open house, and share the news with your neighbors once you are available. This process will help eliminate their anxieties, and they will come to the open house in astonishment. Some may even relocate their parents from across town to your home next door.

Offer an added incentive to your neighbors by extending a discount for their relatives who move in. You can offer a 10 percent discount or waive $500 or even $1,000 a month. If the neighborhood HOA offers resistance, kindly remind them that you're prepared to win with the Fair Housing Act. Pose the following question, "You're not against fair, affordable housing for seniors, are you?" Afterward, extend a 10 percent discount for referrals offered by any HOA member. This incentive will turn lemons into lemonade, enable existing neighbors to refer friends of their friends. This method can help make peace with your HOA and help fill your home quickly. This method will allow you to put solutions in place instead of allowing problems to persist.

RELATIONSHIPS AND REFERRALS

Marketing For New Residents

- •Website
- •Flyers
- •Business Cards
- •Sign In Front
- •Open House

- •Referrals
- •Relationships
- •Hospice
- •Placement Agencies

Marketing residential assisted living homes is a matter of increased exposure, connecting to clients, and getting referrals. Ultimately, most of our business currently comes from referrals. Referrals are based on building relationships. As the owner, that is not necessarily your role, but your manager should be highly engaged in connecting with the community. You could even provide your manager with an expense account of a few hundred dollars a month. These funds allow them to take potential referral sources out to lunch or purchase coffee for referral agencies.

MARKETING TO HOSPICE COMPANIES

Why establish relationships with hospice centers? My first experience with hospice involved my father. He was given a life expectancy of six months. We transitioned him and my mom into our own home. Six months turned into two years. During his final few weeks, hospice visited daily, providing end-of-life care. Now that I am in the business, I understand that these outstanding services were of no charge to me, but they were not free.

We each have an account that is paid for through our taxes. I call that the end-of-life price tag on our lives. As long as there is a portion of this budget remaining and individuals are getting closer to the end of their lives, they may qualify to have some services provided at no cost to them directly. A visiting nurse, a bed, or other needed supplies could be provided. Sometimes, hospice may refer people to us because of the need for 24/7 care, which the hospice themselves do not provide for more than seven days typically. In this scenario, hospice cannot accept referral payments - this is why it's essential to build relationships with hospice companies.

MARKETING STARTS BEFORE
YOU OPEN

On the other hand, placement agencies place seniors in assisted living homes, which is usually a fee-based process.

Despite the expense, it's vital to invite placement agents to visit your home, even during the construction process. Welcome suggestions about things you can consider doing differently. Afterward, they will feel a sense of ownership when they refer potential residents to your home.

THE IMPORTANCE OF MARKETING

Residential assisted living is a rapidly growing business opportunity that attracts many owners, operators, and seniors. Most new owners and operators have minimal experience operating an assisted living business or experience with seniors at all. Marketing is a core concept that can determine whether your business fails or thrives. A marketing plan is an essential marketing tool for every small business. To create an effective strategy, you'll need to start by answering some critical fundamental questions:

- What do you want your assisted living home to accomplish and why?
- What is your target market?
- Who is your competition?

Consider these important questions before taking action. There are ten critical questions every business owner and operator should answer to create an impactful marketing plan.

10 CRITICAL STARTUP QUESTIONS

1. How Will Your Marketing Plan Support Your Business Goals?
2. What Is the Mission You're Trying to Accomplish, and Why?
3. Who Are You Trying to Reach with Your Marketing Activities?
4. Who is your competition, and how do you compare?
5. What Makes Your Business Unique?
6. What Will You Charge, and Why?
7. How Will You Reach Your Target Market?
8. How Much Money Will You Spend, and on What?
9. What Tasks Do You Need to Complete to Reach Your Marketing Goals?
10. What Results Have You Achieved, and Where Can You Improve?

SUCCESS STORIES

"Ultimately, your success is up to you. You can't change your past, but you can create and design your future."

LISTEN ONLINE TO OUR SUCCESSFUL STUDENTS SHARE IN THEIR OWN WORDS

We have a host of video success stories listed on our website at www.RALAcademy.com. You need to know that thousands of former students and associates have had success with starting a RAL business.

Hal of Scottsdale, Arizona, is one of the first students of RAL Academy. When Hal started, we didn't have much support, follow-up, and collection of resources we have available today. We are proud that Hal has achieved success opening his Arizona-based RAL home.

Greg of Fort Collins, Colorado, opened a care home in Fort Collins after his first training in January 2017. It took quite a bit longer for Greg to open his first home, which was due to working with the city government. The RAL training concerning the Fair Housing Act became immediately invaluable. Greg overcame obstacles to secure his financial legacy.

Jeremy of Arizona attended RAL Academy in June 2018 and started with his first home in less than two months after finishing Gene's course. In Jeremy's case, he found an existing home licensed for ten residents. Based on what he learned from RAL Academy, he decided it was a good buy, and he made it his own.

Jeff of Silicon Valley, California, came to the live training event and discovered an opportunity — that he wasn't quite looking for — that wound up working out. What we love about Jeff's story is that he used what he learned from RAL Academy and applied it to a larger facility rather than a residence.

Matt of Murray, Kentucky, runs Southern Grace Assisted Living, located in Kentucky. Southern Grace is in a Frank Lloyd Wright design-inspired home built-in 1975. Southern Grace is a mixed 12-bed home of singles and doubles and could net around $12,000 to $15,000 per month when full, but Matt realistically calculates some vacancy and budgets a net of $10,000 to $12,000 per month consistently.

Join our assisted living family as we work together to provide high-quality care for the rapidly growing senior population in America. We are excited about connecting with you on this intelligent, safe, and secure investment experience in residential assisted living. The Blueprint is a platform where we can all "Do Good and Do Well" together.

Donald and Talinda of St. Louis, Missouri, were motivated by a passion for helping people. Seeing first-hand the issues with their parent's senior living environments, they jumped feet first into residential assisted living. Determined to raise the standards of care and being brought up by a highly entrepreneurial father, Donald had the right mindset to seek out and follow through with the opportunity in assisted living investing.

Their new RAL home is a 12 bedroom, 6,600-square-feet facility that offers adult day services and memory care. The impact of their RAL home in their community has been exciting to watch, and we can't wait to see them expand more homes soon. "Thank you to the RAL Academy. It has been amazing the support we've received from you guys. We wouldn't have been able to make this journey without you," said Donald.

Timothy and Helga of Arizona work as music theory professors and professional musicians. They've had years of experience with single-family rentals but wanted to broaden their investment and create a lasting legacy. They started in residential assisted living by remodeling their own home into a 10-bed, 11-bath RAL facility. The care they provide their residents is focused on holistic health, with advanced nutrition programs, mental and physical exercise, music therapy, and much more. Their most extensive advice for those getting into this business is, "know your why." Find your purpose and embrace it fully.

Mandi of Rhode Island is one of our first RAL Academy students. Mandi and her husband found the opportunity in residential assisted living irresistible. Though initially running into roadblocks with zoning and building regulations, they found their way past obstacles with support from our academy. It's been over three years since they opened their 10-resident RAL home in Rhode Island, and they are genuinely enjoying the fruits of their labor. Mandi's advice to others is, "Continue to ask questions until you get the answers you need to hear."

Justin of Kansas City, Kansas, heard about the RAL Academy through The Real Estate Guys. He was impressed with Gene's approach to investing which prompted him to check out the 1-day training in Kansas City and then the 3-day fast track course in Phoenix, AZ.

With years of real estate experience and attending countless education programs, Justin was drawn to the RAL Blueprint, citing the family-like support in overcoming obstacles as the main difference to other investment training systems. "It's all about the systems," he said. Now, his high-end 12 resident home is up and running and looking at about a 25-percent profitability margin. He is knocking it out of the park, and we couldn't be prouder of him.

Jeff of Tucson, Arizona, was looking for a career change from a corporate aerospace 9-to-5 job. After running the numbers, he looked into real estate and found that he would need to invest in 60 units to match his income. Upon hearing about residential assisted living and the potential to make that same net profit with just one or two single-family homes, it was clear that this was the right choice for investment.

Having attended the RAL Academy 3-day training and completing the home study course, Jeff opened his spacious nine-resident home in Tucson, AZ, and is on his way to filling it. He and his wife aim to expand by opening four RAL homes and eventually helping his employees run their own assisted living homes.

Heather and Kevin of Gilbert, Arizona, had a long-time interest in real estate. Kevin found Gene's RAL Academy system through a real estate podcast. In combination with Heather's passion for her nursing career, his passion pointed to the residential assisted living opportunity as one that just made sense. "Coming out to that 3-day opened our eyes so much to the potential…it was invaluable to us."

Although it took a while to find the right home, they persevered and just took the process one step at a time. They wanted to create the perfect environment. Their 10-resident house is open and operating at total capacity. Now, they are looking to duplicate their efforts and start a second RAL home. Heather and Kevin's had this advice to give to others, "Get the training and seek out advice. It's important to have that support system."

Allyson of Castle Rock, Colorado, is a former public-school teacher who was looking for a solid investment plan for her family. She spent years volunteering in large senior care homes. She heard about residential assisted living as an alternative. "It lined up with my passion and also made a ton of sense," she said. With minimal experience with real estate, health care, or financial planning, Allyson learned everything she needed to open her residential assisted living home by attending the RAL Academy. She also gained assistance available through the platinum support package. She advises anyone getting into this industry to connect and network with people who are already operating RAL homes. She says you should start by asking lots of questions.

Brad and Angie had 15 years of real estate investment experience with rental properties, construction, and property development. Residential assisted living just seemed to be a perfect fit. They looked at this investment opportunity and said, "We need this. Our community needs this."

Based on their experience, one of the most significant benefits they got from the RAL Academy was the support system. Before, people who had been there and done it before were just a phone call away to answer questions and get much-needed advice on project specifics. Despite minor roadblocks along the way, they remained focused. "We always have to keep in mind why we're doing this,"

Brad said. "We want to provide the best quality care we can for seniors."

Ed and Janel of Indiana were looking for an investment opportunity more substantial than rental properties. Life was good with rentals, but it could be a lot better. In addition to the financial motivation, Janel wanted to have a suitable place for her grandma other than the extensive senior care facilities in their area. "I wish there could be a place that's like home," she said. Then this opportunity came along, and "it was meant to be."

With training from the 3-Day Fast Track event, the inner circle network, and continued support from the RAL team, they are progressing quickly with their 16-bedroom RAL home project that will be open soon and provide care to an underserved area highest quality senior care.

Right now, you have a decision to make. Your next step is up to you.

The "Silver Tsunami of Seniors" is coming, and that is undeniable. Whether that Tsunami is a crisis or an opportunity in your life is largely up to you. At the very least, I want to encourage you to own at least 1 RAL home to provide for yourself and your loved ones - this will allow you to pass on a blessing instead of a burden to your kids and grandkids.

At the beginning of the book, I made the statement, "Everyone will get involved in assisted living one way or the other." That's true, and right now, that choice is up to you. Whether you decide to take advantage of the real estate opportunities, the business opportunities, or be a passive investor, it's up to you to take that next step.

I'M IN... WHAT DO I DO NOW?

Get started by visiting us at <u>RALAcademy.com</u> or call us at 480-704-3065.

BUILDING A LEGACY

*"They say you shouldn't judge a book by its cover.
That may be true.
I say you should judge a man by his family and
friends. Welcome to my family."*

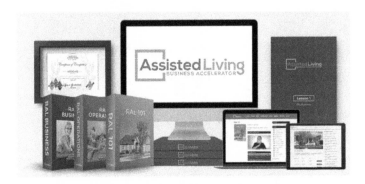

THE MAKING OF THE SILVER TSUNAMI
OF SENIORS

Gene Guarino has been an entrepreneur his entire life. He was a professional musician as a teenager and started his first official business at 16. He purchased his 1st residential property at the age of 18 and his 1st commercial property at 25. Now, with over 40 years of experience in real estate investing and with over two dozen businesses to date, Gene is focused on just one thing, Residential Assisted Living.

It was 1998 when Gene first realized the tremendous business opportunities resulting from the unstoppable Silver Tsunami of seniors. It wasn't until his mother needed assistance that he committed to getting into the industry and becoming a part of the solution. That's when it became more than just a financial opportunity – it became personal. As a result, Gene got started in residential assisted living in 2013. *"When we needed to find a place for mom to call home, that's when residential assisted living became personal for me."*

Today Gene and his family not only own and operate RAL homes. They invest in other homes and train others on the steps needed so they can also do it. He's the founder of the "AL Family" group of companies, including the Residential Assisted Living Academy, The RAL National Association, The AL Network, and Family Legacy Homes. Live Training Registration

THE RESIDENTIAL ASSISTED LIVING ACADEMY

RALA is a private (non-accredited) assisted living education company that teaches everything from A-Z about meeting the rising demand for senior housing. Guarino's 3-day fast track empowers students to support themselves by achieving true financial independence. Guarino owns and operates RAL homes and has students all across the country that are also benefiting from this lucrative niche in business and real estate. He travels internationally, facilitating seminars and business teachings that focus on his model/blueprint for assisted living. He helps individuals generate cash flow through passive activity focused on owning and operating RAL homes. The RAL Academy's motto is "*Do Good and Do Well.*" Click Here To Learn More About the Assisted Living Webinar

PREPARING FOR THE SILVER TSUNAMI OF SENIORS

The unstoppable Silver Tsunami of Seniors comprises about 77 million baby boomers, with 10,000 people turning 65 daily and 4,000 seniors a day turning 85. About 70 percent of these people will need assisted living at some point. Guarino is also co-author of Investing in Senior Housing and author of self-published books, *Virtual Entrepreneur* and *Cash for Kids* (Volume I & II). During a 2016 symposium at Harvard University School of Business, the self-taught assisted living entrepreneur shared how to turn a single-family home into a monthly $5,000-$15,000 cash flow. Visit the Residential Assisted Living Academy on Facebook at: https://www.facebook.com/ResidentialAssistedLivingAcademy

His new book, *The Silver Tsunami of Seniors,* will help you start your own RAL business and gain financial freedom. To truly understand who Gene Guarino is, you have to understand better the "Why" behind his purpose and passion.

WHO IS GENE GUARINO?

A LEGACY FOR MOM

I was at a Real Estate conference many years ago, and the speaker was talking about opportunities in real estate. He spoke about how the baby boomers were driving the world's economy and how "Residential assisted living was going to be the best place to be." Immediately after his presentation, I ran up to him and asked him to tell me more. He replied, "I can't. I've never done it; I'm just telling you; you should do it." Have you ever shared a similar experience where the guru in the front of the room told you what to do, yet they weren't even doing it themselves?

I own, operate, and invest in residential assisted living homes. When I first heard about residential assisted living homes, I couldn't find anyone to teach me how to do it. I searched for someone to show me, but I couldn't find anyone, as previously explained in my introduction:

In the end, I knew what I had to do, get committed, and take action.

As time went on, life got busy, and my interest faded until I watched my mother suffering – her name is Marie. Mom invested her entire life caring for others. She raised seven children and taught school before retiring to Florida with our dad. During my dad's health challenges, she was his caregiver until he passed. Afterward, mom cared for her elderly mother until my grandmother also passed. During the last few years of mom's life, she started forgetting to take her meds, skipping dinner, and suffering from memory loss. After she experienced a fall, things took a turn for the worse – Mom needed full-time assisted living care.

These trying times were difficult experiences for our family. For the first time in her life, at age 86, she needed someone to take care of her. It wasn't long before my siblings and I realized how miserable many assisted living choices were.

That's when my Big Why become clear – it was suddenly fueled with passion. I vowed to create an excellent assisted living home where I'd be proud to have my mother live. I wrote down my goal, and soon after, my Big Why became a reality. Now, my passion is to spread *The Silver Tsunami of Seniors* across the country for high-quality assisted living in a residential setting.

Residential Assisted Living Academy provides a different kind of eye-opening experience. As the owner of RAL homes and as an educator with a passion to teacher and a mission to accomplish, I provide students with a 3-day fast-track course. My fast-track training includes live tours and interactive sessions that explore everything from A-Z in residential assisted living. Our nationwide team of industry experts offers professional training and support with decades of combined experience. We've helped owners, operators, and businesses avoid losses incurred by trial and error. (Visit www.RALAcademy.com for more information about the 3-day fast-track training). My challenges and successes have prepared me to teach others how to avoid the same mistakes and disappointments I had to endure. We provide the fast-track to your success.

RALA - WHERE IT ALL BEGAN

I remember receiving the phone call, "Mom fell, you need to get here now!" I was 2000 miles away. It was a late afternoon, and the sun was setting, even though it wasn't even 4 p.m. yet. I was on a plane and breaking through the clouds descending on my way to see Mom. Swirling snow flurries raced by the window of the aircraft. Winters in upstate New York are primarily gray and cold. I never seemed to notice when I was a kid. Now that I live in Arizona, east coast winters seem even more frigid, grayer and harsher every time I visit. Learn more about Gene Guarino's story on YouTube at: https://www.youtube.com/user/Yoitsmetv

We have a ritual when we land at the Albany airport. We always take a picture of the giant wooden sphere covered in handles and hooks, located in the corridor between the gates and baggage claim. This time, it was different. While taking the picture, memories flooded my mind about my childhood growing up in upstate New York.

I come from a big family with seven kids who shared two committed parents. My parents stayed committed for more than 50 years throughout all the challenges, successes, failures, and difficulties. They were great examples. Now that I've been married for more than 30 years, with four kids and grandkids of my own, I have a better understanding of commitment and how rare it is in today's world.

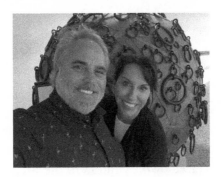

After retrieving our bags from the carousel, we picked up our rental car. As a teen, driving in the freshly fallen snow was fun. Now, I'd rather "eat" donuts than "do" donuts while driving on slippery roads. We managed slowly to make our way up the Northway to exit 8, heading towards my mom's home. Although it was a short drive, I was nervously anxious to see her. It had only been a few months since my last visit, but it felt far too long. The older I get, the more value I place on how precious time is. Time seems to be moving faster every day.

The older I get, the more time I spend gazing into the wondrous night sky at God's creation. Time is racing against life, and it makes me wonder, "How many more full moons will I get?" Entrepreneurs can learn more about the RAL Academy on Twitter at: https://twitter.com/ralacademy

THE BEGINNING OF THE END

I knew that my time with mom was coming to an end. I didn't know when – we never do. We arrived at mom's home and walked through the front door. This time everything felt different. Mom didn't greet us with her usual colossal hug and warm welcome. This time, she was sitting in her chair in the front room. Mom had fallen and cracked a couple of ribs days before my visit, and that chair had become her bed. As a result, there was no colossal hug that only mom could give. Join the webinar to learn more about residential assisted living: ral101.com.

I knew the pain she was experiencing physically restricted her from embracing me with her smothering mother's hug. Yet, we still knew that she was happy to see us. So, I bent over and gave her a little kiss on the forehead and a gentle hug. Upon looking around, I noticed that life had changed for mom. She wasn't as sweet-smelling as she usually was, and the room was messier than usual, even for mom. She wasn't a hoarder, but she kept things within hands reach if you know what I mean. There was always something nearby that she wanted to use for show-and-telling or a gift to give. It could be a newspaper article, a recipe, or another personal treasure that she was sure we needed to see or have. It was all a part of what made mom special to us all – we continue to laugh about that today. When we get together as a family, these are some of the things we reminisce about concerning mom and dad. I didn't know at the time, but this visit was the beginning of the end for mom. Click the following link to learn more about the assisted living home study course training program: https://ralacademy.online.

YOU'VE GOT 6 MONTHS TO LIVE

Ten years before that visit, dad had already passed away. His death is somewhat complicated to explain. A procedure followed a heart problem to unblock plaque that traveled to his brain, which caused a stroke, resulting in a rare fungus.

It went something like that. I'm not a medical professional, and I avoid doctors as much as possible unless I play poker, smoke a cigar, or enjoy a glass of red wine with them. Either way, I don't have a lot of doctors as close friends. Schedule a discovery before getting involved in the assisted living industry by clicking the link below: ral101.com.

The human body is incredible, but it can only handle so much. I don't know what I would think if I were to get that news today. "**Mr. Guarino, I am sorry to inform you that you only have six months to live.** I suggest that you get your affairs in order and say your goodbyes." Perhaps I'd start thinking of things I've always wanted to do and places I hoped to travel to worldwide. Suddenly, my bucket list became a priority list. Maybe I'd say, "Why did I waste so much time and energy on the small and unimportant things in life?" It's easy to speculate, especially when you're healthy. **We all have an "expiration date," we don't know what it is yet.**

However, when you know your rapidly approaching expiration date in advance, your story is likely to change. With only six months to live, reality suddenly changed for dad and our entire family.

GOD'S WAITING ROOM

Mom and dad were living in Florida, where all good New Yorkers report when they retire. Some people say that 'Florida is God's waiting room." The joke is that people retire and then move to Florida, buy a retirement home, purchase a burial plot, and wait life out. Unfortunately, for many, there seems to be some truth to that. Currently, the Silver Tsunami of Seniors is hitting the shores hard in Florida and other warm-weather states. It's unstoppable. **Most people fail to prepare for what's coming their way as they age.**

MY WIFE, MONA, IS INCREDIBLE

After we heard the news about dad, we invited mom and dad to move in with us in our home in Upstate, NY. Mona was the one that suggested it. Her selfless and kind gesture was a gift to them and me. Six months isn't long in the scope of things, but most spouses aren't willing to have their in-laws move into their homes. Mona didn't miss a beat. She is such an amazing hostess, whether it's an evening party or a long-term stay, she makes accommodations. My family and I couldn't thank Mona enough.

We were so happy to have them live with us. We had no idea how long our parents would have to stay in our Ballston Lake, New York home. Country Knolls was the name of the development, and Mona's family lived about a mile away in the same neighborhood. It was a blessing to see Les and Claire, my in-laws, regularly - they live in Florida now. We do get to see them from time to time, but it seems like it's never often enough.

Mona and I both come from families with seven children, and we are both the fifth child amongst our siblings. Some things are meant to be. Both were "good catholic families" that held up their end of the bargain by having prominent families. I love Les and Claire, and they have come to love and appreciate me as well. Although, when I asked Les for his daughter's hand in marriage, he cried like a baby – and they were not tears of joy. That is an entirely different story for another time.

Before mom and dad moved in, we had to make some household arrangements. Our home was a raised ranch, and we had a rental apartment in the lower half, which generated income. I'd purchased my first property at age 18. So, by this time, I gained a lot of experience in the real estate and investing industry. Our tenant's lease was coming up for renewal, and we informed them about the situation. We wanted to spend as much time as we could with my dad. Therefore, we would not be renewing their lease. They understood, and Mom and Dad moved in soon after.

THE POWER OF FAMILY

We were grateful every day, and six months turned into two years for my dad. When Mom and Dad moved into our home, they spent a lot of time with the grandkids. I believe this environment helped Dad live well beyond expectations. As I reminisce, I can see how that experience was a precursor to my destiny in residential assisted living. My mom served as the caregiver 24 hours a day, seven days a week – Dad didn't need a nursing home, but he did need assistance. If he were in a sizeable commercial building packed with seniors, I don't think he would have lived nearly as long in a "Big Box" facility. Being surrounded by family is essential for everyone, regardless of your age. Read weekly blogs about assisted living at: https://residentialassistedlivingacademy.com/blog/.

"DOING GOOD" COMES IN MANY FORMS

This motto is our mission of helping others while making money in the process. Unfortunately, there is an epidemic of loneliness in our world today. Providing seniors with care, comfort, and a safe home to live in with a community of peers, is all a part of "Doing Good and Doing Well."

During those two years, we spent as much time as we could with mom and dad. Although we still wanted them to have their own space. Looking back, I wish I had spent even more time with them but isn't that always the case?

In life, typically, we don't regret the things we do – it's the things that we don't do that we tend to regret. That is one of many life lessons that have served me well. As a result, today, I say "yes" to many things, especially when it comes to spending time with the family.

I make decisions quickly so that I can move forward faster. Life is short. Since we all have an unknown expiration date, love the people around you, live your life fully, and avoid regrets. Having mom and dad living with us was a huge blessing. The farther that memory fades into the distant past, the more I realize just how much of a benefit it was. Of course, some days were better than others, but overall, it was a fantastic time, and I am so thankful that they were there. As dad was getting closer to the end, hospice workers and volunteers came to the house to help. At that time, I knew nothing about hospice. These hospice workers seemed to be sent by God. We were incredibly blessed and appreciative to have their help.

A BETTER PLACE? ABSOLUTELY!

"Dad died." Those words are packed with a powerful punch no matter who says it, and regardless of where you are when you hear it. It's the kind of a punch in the gut that takes your breath away – those are heavy words. Even though he'd been given more time than expected, the loss is no less painful. I remember reflecting over his body at his funeral and realizing that "he" wasn't there.

Dad was clearly in a better place. I wasn't upset because I knew that his spirit had left that body, and his spirit is his true essence – he is free. All I was looking at was the "meat suit" he occupied here on earth. God is incredible. I am sure that God is in control. Thoughts about Dad came to mind every day until Mom died. Once they were together again, my heart was settled. We are spirits residing in the flesh for a short season on earth.

PASSION FOR TEACHING AND A LOVE FOR LEARNING

Dad was an inquisitive man, constantly learning about something. If he had the internet at his fingertips, like we do today, there is no telling what he would have researched. He loved traveling after retiring from his teaching career. He loved to travel so much that he started a travel division at a local bus company that transformed their business and changed lives.

Investing in family vacations is one of the most important lessons I learned from Dad. Spending time with your family and friends is invaluable. I always knew that my mom was an entrepreneur at heart, but Dad had it in him. Dad was a college professor for over 30 years. He earned his Ph.D. in education and served as president of the reading department at SUNY Albany. He loved teaching teachers how to teach. Some people train because they can. Great teachers do it to share their love of learning with others. Dad was a great teacher, it was his passion, and he passed his passion for teaching onto me. My dad died at age 70, far too soon, but forever loved.

MOM'S NEXT ASSIGNMENT

After Dad passed away, my mother took on her next assignment. My grandmother needed help. By this time, grandma was over 100 years old. Mom's side of the family has longevity in their DNA, without a doubt. My grandfather lived to be an older man, taking long walks to the country club and smoking cigars daily. Now, I share the same desire for long walks and cigars. I'll never forget his prickly kiss on the cheek when we would visit him in Connecticut. I wonder if my mustache is as prickly to my grandkids. Perhaps they'll talk about it when I'm gone.

Mom moved in with my grandmother to take care for her full time. Since Mom was a nurse by profession, she was well-trained to care of others. She lived with her mother to the very end. They eventually moved grandma's bed downstairs into the dining room - this prevented her from having to climb the stairs to her bedroom. She lived to be 104 years old. Her funeral was a high-spirited celebration of life for our entire family.

RANDOM MEMORIES

I remember grandma paying the neighborhood boys a quarter to make me do sit-ups. She used to say I was too "husky" – that may have been true. They were paid well when I visited, but it didn't help. Grandma was a good cook, and her Toll House Chocolate Chip Cookies were well worth the 3-hour drive from upstate New York. Maybe it was all the extra butter and sugar she added that made them so addictive. Mom was also a great cook, although she seemed only to have five recipes that she made on a regular rotation:

1. Potato Lasagna or Homemade Pierogi,
2. Crispy Macaroni and Cheese,
3. Stuffed Peppers,
4. Beans and Hotdogs, and
5. Friday Fish Fries.

Remember, we were a good Catholic family; my six brothers and sisters and I were well fed. Back then, things were different. As a college professor, at the height of Dad's career, he earned less than $40,000. His income was enough for us to live comfortably, but it wasn't enough for many extra things that we all take for granted today. The only restaurant I remember is McDonald's. The nearest McDonald's was about 15 miles away, and we only went once a month. It's funny what you remember from your childhood – the events, the moments, and the experiences.

My wife, Mona, is an incredible cook, as any guest in our home will attest. She will see a picture on the cover of a magazine, get the recipe, and make it to perfection without hesitation. Mona loves making desserts. She once owned and operated her cake decorating business called

MonaBella Cakes. So, the very thing that Grandma paid dearly to rid me of, I am now doomed to experience due to Mona's amazingly talent of cooking. It looks like I will be husky forever, but I accept that cross in life.

After grandma passed away, mom moved into a town-home located a few miles away from our childhood home in Clifton Park, New York. I still remember the phone number to the (landline) house phone. It rings to the local cab company now. I sometimes test it for fun. I drive by the old house once in a while and reminisce about our childhood adventures. That house seems small now, but it felt much more significant when I was growing up. Funny how perspectives change. I have fond memories of sharing a room with my brothers. Well, some of those memories aren't so fond. I remember when mom took a roll of masking tape to divide the room into two halves because we were constantly fighting one another.

Ahhh, those were the days. I remember finally getting my room when my older siblings moved out. I remember when Pete Mallia, who owned a pool company, gave us an above-ground swimming pool for the backyard. I remember learning how to play the drums in the basement and driving my parents' crazy in the process. My first jobs were cutting the neighbor's grass in the summer, raking their autumn leaves, and shoveling the winter snow from their driveways. I even remember my first house party when my parents were away and the first time I damaged their car. That house reminds me of many of my "first" experiences.

The current owners of my childhood home probably wonder why a strange man with a white beard parks in front of their house from time to time. What might strike their curiosity is when I start taking pictures before I pull away.

No matter what your next assignment is in life, you will never forget your humble beginnings. Those memories are a culmination of who you'll become as life goes on.

A SUDDEN SHIFT

The night I received a call from my sister is seared into my memory. She informed me that Mom fell out of her bed. My sister, Anne, had been living with my mother for a couple of years. It was good for them both to have each other, but I am sure they drove one another crazy from time to time. Once Anne told me what happened, I instinctively knew that it was the beginning of a new chapter in Mom's life. Mom used to do anything within her power to help others, and now SHE needed help.

DECISIONS HAD TO BE MADE

1. Who would take care of her?
2. Would we hire a caregiver from the outside to come into her home?
3. Is it time to consider putting her into a home?

I felt guilty even thinking about putting Mom into any home besides my own. These questions scared us all.

IT WAS THE LAST THING WE ALL WANTED TO DO
1. What would that look like?
2. How much would it cost?
3. Where would the right home be?

The questions were coming fast, but the answers took time. It was a serious matter that happened so suddenly. Mom needed help, and it was time to do the right thing.

By this time, we were living in Phoenix, Arizona. We moved after Dad died because we felt that God called us to help plant a church. We were right – we heard his voice, and we followed that call. Our families in upstate New York didn't want us to relocate. We both have six siblings who were all starting families. We would host family gatherings for almost everything, and even birthday parties had 20-30 people. Our home was the center of many of those parties and gatherings. When both sides of our family came together, it was a huge event.

God spoke to our hearts. We sold our home and moved to Arizona with five other families. Upon arrival, we planted the church. It's 25-years later, and a lot has changed. However, our commitment to God is still the same. We were blessed with an incredible journey when we moved to Arizona. I was traveling and teaching others how to invest in real estate, trade stocks, and start their businesses. I've always been a teacher at heart, thanks to Dad. I am also an entrepreneur, thanks to Mom. When I got that fateful call from my sister, Anne, it was during one of my trips.

I immediately made plans to see Mom. When I walked through the front door, seeing my mother suffer due to her fall was a real wake-up call. Her pain pierced my heart.

BUSINESS OR PERSONAL?

From a business perspective, I'd heard about the opportunities with the aging baby boomer generation. Although, when I first heard about it twenty years early, the timing was far off. I am a baby boomer, and it wasn't me that needed help – it was my mom. The course of events expected to take place decades into the future was hitting me in the face right at that very moment. Right now, it isn't the baby boomers who need assisted living; it's their parents. When the boomers get to that point in life, the silver tsunami will be a full-on crisis. For business-minded individuals, it will be a full-on opportunity of a lifetime.

WE COULDN'T FIND WHAT WE WERE LOOKING FOR

The senior communities that we visited were BIG and depressing. The options for mom were not appealing. They certainly didn't feel at home. Some were hospitals converted, and others were institutional-style buildings occupied by 80 or more residents. These buildings were comprised of large campuses that segregated seniors into isolation. These facilities were detached from traditional neighborhoods – and that didn't feel right either.

There were only two residential homes in neighborhoods within a 50-mile radius in our upstate New York Community. They were bigger homes used for residential assisted living, but they were not well designed, and they were poorly kept. The one "good" home was fully occupied. They had a waiting list, but so did the "bad" house. It was packed, too. We were experiencing a crisis, and we needed a solution. I needed help, and I knew instantly that millions of people would need the same help soon. That's when I made a vow to create a home that I would be proud to have my mother live.

THE BIRTH OF THE RESIDENTIAL ASSISTED LIVING ACADEMY

Since we couldn't find the right home for my mom, I vowed to create it. I set out to create a home that I would be proud to have my mother reside. I knew that if I did that, it would attract others, too. I was right. That vow was the first step in the process of getting into the assisted living business. I saw the need first-hand, and it became very personal. I had a real strong reason to do it, which became my "Big Why" behind my commitment. Let's face it, it's easy to talk about doing something, but starting a business takes a lot more than talking. You have to get committed and accept the following steps.

I researched opening a home in upstate New York, where my mother was living. It was possible, but I didn't know how to get started. Starting the process from beginning to completion while living more than 2000 miles away was going to be a difficult task. So, I made no excuses and proceeded with my plans to start a quality care home in Arizona. There were no classes or training academies teaching students how to create residential assisted living homes. I couldn't find anyone willing or able to show me how to do it.

EVERYONE I MET DOING RAL
FIT INTO ONE OF THREE CATEGORIES:

1. Willing to share, but not good at teaching,
2. Doing it unsuccessfully and tried to talk me out of it,
3. Successful, but too busy or unwilling to share.

In the end, I knew what I had to do.

I had to get committed and take action.

I had a vision of what I wanted for Mom, and since I couldn't find it, I created it. I wanted to own the industry and provide a great home with quality care. I didn't want to work in the business daily. I couldn't find the model of residential assisted living I wanted. That's when I knew that I needed to create it myself, so I did.

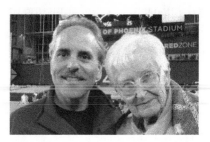

I am fortunate in many ways. My mom lived with my sister, Anne, for over ten years. Toward the end, she moved into my sister, Chris's home, with her family. Thankfully, Anne, Chris, and her family loved and cared for Mom until the end. We had caregivers that came to the home and provided some assistance along the way. However, both Anne, Chris, and her family offered tremendous love and cared for Mom. Near the end, hospice also provided some care. By the time I'd opened my first home, mom was well into the final inning of her game. She left a lasting legacy through her kids and grandchildren. Mom never got to see my homes in person, but she did in spirit – I'm sure of that.

THE BLUEPRINT FOR RESIDENTIAL ASSISTED LIVING

There are millions of seniors right now that will need assistance. Studies show that about 70 percent of them will need help with their Activities of Daily Living (ADLs) for an average of 3.5 years. According to AARP, nearly 90 percent of seniors want to stay at home and live out their lives. Unfortunately, many of them will need help daily. They will need a place to live and someone to take care of them. That is either a crisis or an opportunity, depending on which side of the coin you choose to focus.

I decided since no one was willing or able to teach me how to start, own and operate a residential assisted living homes, I'd figure it out on my own. I do not recommend this lengthy process for others. When there is no option, you have to do what you have to do. What I learned through that experience cost me hundreds of thousands of dollars in mistakes, lost revenue, and missed opportunities. It was difficult, painful, and expensive. I only wish I had someone that had done it before to show me how. That would have saved me many growing pains and lessons I paid a high price to learn.

The good news for you is, I've successfully done it. Now I'm teaching others how to do it. The Residential Assisted Living Academy was created to give individuals the knowledge, resources, and encouragement needed to start their business faster, more efficiently, and effectively.

IN MEMORIAM

Gene had over 30 years experience in real estate investing and business and shifted his focus to just one thing… investing in the mega-trend of senior assisted housing.

Having trained tens of thousands of investors/entrepreneurs over the past 25 years, he built the Residential Assisted Living Academy to specialize in helping others take advantage of this mega-trend opportunity.

Gene passed away in October of 2021 and leaves behind an incredible legacy; one that is carried on by his family, these companies, and the countless people he impacted."

Learn more about Gene by visiting: https://residentialassistedlivingacademy.com/meet-gene/

REFERENCES AND RESOURCE LINKS

Events
https://residentialassistedlivingacademy.com/
live-training-registration/

Discovery Call
https://go.oncehub.com/RALAcademyDiscoveryCall

Webinar
ral101.com

RNC
www.ralnationalconvention.com

RALNA
www.ralna.org

RALA Facebook
https://www.facebook.com/
ResidentialAssistedLivingAcademy

RALNA Facebook Group
https://www.facebook.com/groups/ralna

RALA YouTube
https://www.youtube.com/user/Yoitsmetv

RALA Twitter
https://twitter.com/ralacademy

RALA Instagram
https://www.instagram.com/ralacademy/

RALA Blogs
https://residentialassistedlivingacademy.com/blog/

RALA Home Study Course Training Program Page
https://residentialassistedlivingacademy.com/
home-study-course/

Pitch Masters Academy
www.pitchmastersacademy.com

Memory Care Training, Fill Your Home Fast Training,
Home Tours Training
https://ralacademy.online